Diagnosis and Management of Female Obstructive Genital Malformations

Lan Zhu • Felix Wong • Sara Y. Brucker
Editors

Diagnosis and Management of Female Obstructive Genital Malformations

Springer

Editors
Lan Zhu
Department of Obstetrics and Gynecology
Peking Union Medical College Hospital
Beijing, China

Felix Wong
Department of Obstetrics and Gynecology
Liverpool Hospital
Liverpool, NSW, Australia

Sara Y. Brucker
Department of Obstetrics and Gynecology
Tubingen University Hospital
Tübingen, Germany

ISBN 978-981-19-6758-0 ISBN 978-981-19-6759-7 (eBook)
https://doi.org/10.1007/978-981-19-6759-7

This Springer imprint is published by the registered company Springer Nature Singapore Pte Ltd.
The registered company address is: 152 Beach Road, #21-01/04 Gateway East, Singapore 189721, Singapore

Contents

Part I
Introduction

Chapter 1
Overview of Obstructive Uterovaginal Anomalies

Na Chen and Lan Zhu

Abstract Obstructive uterovaginal anomalies include malformations in which the uterus has functional endometrium but is partially or completely obstructed at or below the uterus. These malformations may lead to partial or complete obstruction in the lower female genital tract and cause substantial negative impact on the physical and psychological health of adolescent girls. Accurate diagnosis and proper treatment are essential for relieving symptoms and long-term prognosis.

Keywords Congenital female genital tract malformations · Reconstruction surgery

Obstructive uterovaginal anomalies include malformations in which the uterus has functional endometrium but is partially or completely obstructed at or below the uterus. The obstruction may result in the obstruction of menstrual blood and corresponding physical or reproductive dysfunction. The main symptoms associated with obstructive uterovaginal anomalies include post-pubertal amenorrhea, dysmenorrhea, pelvic pain, recurrent vaginal drainage, infertility, or obstructed labor [1]. Evaluation of patients with suspected obstructive uterovaginal anomalies requires complete history taking and physical and imaging examinations. Accurate diagnosis is essential for proper management. A good clinical outcome depends on complete disease evaluation, adequate preoperative counseling, thorough surgical intervention, and long-term postoperative management.

N. Chen · L. Zhu (✉)
Department of Obstetrics and Gynecology, Peking Union Medical College Hospital, Peking Union Medical College, Chinese Academy of Medical Sciences, Beijing, China

L. Zhu et al. (eds.), *Diagnosis and Management of Female Obstructive Genital Malformations*, https://doi.org/10.1007/978-981-19-6759-7_1

1.1 Classifications

According to the different sites and degree of the obstruction, obstructive uterovaginal anomalies can be divided into the following categories [2].

1. Obstructive Uterine Malformation
   - 1.1 Mayer-Rokintansky-Kuster-Hauser syndrome with functional endometrium
   - 1.2 Unicornuate uterus complicated with rudimentary horn and uterus with functional endometrium
   - 1.3 Robert uterus
   - 1.4 Accessory cavitated uterine mass
2. Obstructive Cervical Malformations
   - 2.1 Cervical aplasia
   - 2.2 Cervical dysplasia (including fragmentation, fibrous cord, atresia, external os obstruction) with or without bifid uterine anomalies
3. Obstructive Vaginal Malformations
   - 3.1 Vaginal atresia
     - 3.1.1 Partial vaginal atresia
     - 3.1.2 Complete vaginal atresia
   - 3.2 Oblique vaginal septum syndrome (also known as Herlyn-Werner--Wunderlich syndrome) [3]
     - 3.2.1 Subtype I—without holes
     - 3.2.2 Subtype II—with holes
     - 3.2.3 Subtype III—without holes combined with a cervical fistula
     - 3.2.4 Subtype IV—with ipsilateral cervical atresia
   - 3.3 Transverse vaginal septum
     - 3.3.1 Perforated transverse vaginal septum
     - 3.3.2 Non-perforated transverse vaginal septum
4. Obstructive Hymenal Malformations
   - 4.1 Imperforate hymen
   - 4.2 Micropore hymen
5. Obstructive Vulvar Malformations
   - 5.1 Labial fusion—primary and secondary
6. Obstructive Cloacal Malformations
   - 6.1 Single perineal orifice
   - 6.2 Common urogenital orifice

1.2 Symptoms

1. Abdominal pain: The most common symptom caused by obstruction is abdominal pain [1], The pain may occur in a cyclic, irregular, or persistent manner.
2. Menstrual abnormalities: The most common menstrual abnormalities are primary amenorrhea combined with or without pain. Special attention should be paid to exclude possible uterovaginal anomalies for adolescent females who present with combined primary amenorrhea and abdominal pain. In women with symptoms such as irregular vaginal bleeding and pain, the possibility of partial obstructive uterovaginal anomalies should be considered. Patients with spontaneous perforation of the transverse vaginal septum may suddenly experience massive menstrual bleeding.
3. Purulent vaginal discharge: Patients with partial obstructive uterovaginal anomalies may have purulent vaginal discharge that could be caused by abnormal vaginal bleeding or retrograde pelvic infection.
4. Dyspareunia: Patients with a transverse vaginal septum or imperforate hymen or vaginal atresia may complain of dyspareunia or heavy vaginal bleeding due to the tearing of the septum during intercourse.
5. Infertility: Patients usually present with symptoms of genital obstruction during adolescence, and few patients present solely for infertility.
6. Obstructed labor: Few patients with incomplete transverse or oblique vaginal septum can present with obstetric obstruction at the time of delivery.
7. Ectopic pregnancy: Functional rudimentary uterine horn pregnancies may persist into the second trimester and cause life-threatening intra-abdominal bleeding once ruptured.
8. Other associated symptoms include urinary frequency, dysuria, hematuria, and urinary retention. Patients with lower vaginal obstruction may experience tenesmus due to compression of the rectum by an enlarged genital mass.

1.3 Physical Examinations

1. *General examination:* Secondary sex characteristics, such as the presence of laryngeal knots, breasts, pubic hair, and armpit hair development, should be examined to exclude abnormalities. A thorough examination should be performed to determine whether there are combined abnormalities of the kidneys, spine, heart, anorectal opening, trachea-esophagus, limbs, and other systemic development. Abdominal examination may confirm abdominal tenderness or enlarged masses due to blood accumulation in the vagina or uterus caused by obstruction.
2. *Vaginal examination:* Vaginal examination of the female genital tract is essential to differentiate imperforate hymen from labial fusion, genitourinary sinus retention, vaginal septum, or distal vaginal atresia.

3. *Anal examination:* In adolescents, the anal examination is less painful than a vaginal examination and can help confirm the presence of the cervix and assess the distance between the accumulated vaginal blood and the perineum in patients with vaginal atresia or hymenal obstruction.

1.4 Auxiliary Examinations

1.4.1 Radiographic Examinations

1. Ultrasonography: Ultrasonography is the most used and effective radiographic examination. Pelvic ultrasound is recommended for patients with amenorrhea, periodic, intermittent, or persistent abdominal pain. For adolescents who are not sexually active, transrectal or transperineal ultrasonography is preferred. Pelvic endometriosis or adenomyosis should be screened for patients with obstructive uterovaginal anomalies.
2. Magnetic resonance imaging (MRI): For patients with unclear pelvic ultrasound diagnosis or complex genital tract anomalies, pelvic MRI is recommended. MRI is superior in identifying the presence of uterine remnants, endometrium, cervix, proximal vagina, and vaginal blood accumulation [4].

1.4.2 Laboratory Tests

1. Chromosome karyotyping: Most patients with obstructive uterovaginal anomalies have normal female karyotypes (46, XX).
2. Female sex hormone and serum Anti-Müllerian Hormone (AMH) level: The ovarian development and function are normal in patients with obstructive uterovaginal anomalies, so female sex hormone and serum AMH levels are within the normal range in these patients.
3. Serum CA125 level: Elevated serum CA125 levels help diagnose concomitant endometriosis or adenomyosis in patients with obstructive anomalies.

1.5 Treatment

Principles of treatment for patients with obstructive uterovaginal anomalies are as follows:

1. Obstructive uterovaginal anomalies are not surgical emergencies [1]. It is best to be diagnosed and treated by experienced gynecologists familiar with the

treatment of such diseases. Referral to medical institutions with extensive experience in diagnosing and treating such diseases is highly recommended.

2. The first surgical correction of obstructive anomalies is very important for the prognosis of these patients. For medical institutions with insufficient experience in treating such diseases, gynecological examination under anesthesia may be performed only as the first treatment. Simple obstructed vaginal incision and drainage should not be the only procedure performed, for it can cause a high incidence of ascending infection and sepsis and may also complicate subsequent standardized surgical treatment. Genital reconstructive surgery should be performed at the same time as the incision. The first surgery is essential for the patency of the reconstructive genital tract and stenosis prevention.
3. Indications for emergency management include urinary retention, severe abdominal pain, and ascending infection. Under an emergency, a urinary catheter should be placed to relieve symptoms if the patient develops acute urinary retention. Stool-softening medications should be given to patients with concomitant bowel difficulties. Analgesia should also be given to patients to control severe abdominal pain. Broad-spectrum antibiotics should be given for infection, and the patient should be urgently referred to a medical facility with extensive experience for further diagnosis and treatment of genital tract abscesses and ascending infections.
4. For patients who are not prepared for correction surgery in the short term, hormone suppression therapy should be used to prevent menstruation, reduce abdominal pain, protect uterine and ovarian function, as well as reduce the occurrence of endometriosis and adenomyosis, and improve the quality of life. For adolescent patients, menstrual suppression can postpone surgery until the patient is psychologically mature to understand the diagnosis of the disease and accept postoperative vaginal dilation therapy. Patients can also actively participate in the formulation of treatment plans and timing.

1.6 Postoperative Care

1. Postoperative use of vaginal molds is necessary for patients with high risks of postoperative stenosis or reobstruction. The time of mold expansion or placement needs to be individually formulated.
2. Adequate communication with the patient and her family about the diseases and treatment, as well as psychological support: Patients and their families do not have much knowledge about the development of the female genital tract, so educating them about anatomy and menstrual physiology can increase their understanding of the disease. Experienced gynecologists will fully communicate with adolescent patients to prepare her psychologically for the surgery, learn self-care after the surgery, and actively cooperate with doctors for surgical decision-making and postoperative management.

1.7 Long-Term Follow-Up

Patients with obstructive uterovaginal anomalies are at high risk of postoperative infection, restenosis, pelvic endometriosis, and adenomyosis. Postoperative patients with obstructive anomalies should be followed closely and for a long time, and postoperative fertility-related issues should be addressed proactively [5].

In conclusion, a complete disease evaluation, adequate knowledge of the developmental anomalies, experienced surgical intervention, adequate preoperative counseling, and comprehensive long-term postoperative management are essential for optimal outcomes in patients with obstructive uterovaginal anomalies. Next, this book provides a breakdown of the diagnosis and treatment of different types of obstructive uterovaginal anomalies.

References

1. Management of acute obstructive uterovaginal anomalies: ACOG Committee Opinion, Number 779. Obstet Gynecol. 2019;133(6):e363–71. https://doi.org/10.1097/AOG.0000000000003281.
2. Chinese expert consensus on the diagnosis and treatment of obstructive uterine and vaginal dysplasia. Chin J Obstet Gynecol Pediatr. 2021;56(11):746–52. https://doi.org/10.3760/CMA.J.CN112141-20210824-00466.
3. Zhu L, Chen N, Tong JL, Wang W, Zhang L, Lang JH. New classification of Herlyn-Werner-Wunderlich syndrome. Chin Med J. 2015;128(2):222–5. https://doi.org/10.4103/0366-6999.149208.
4. Saleem SN. MR imaging diagnosis of uterovaginal anomalies: current state of the art. Radiographics. 2003;23(5):e13. https://doi.org/10.1148/rg.e13.
5. Joki-Erkkilä MM, Heinonen PK. Presenting and long-term clinical implications and fecundity in females with obstructing vaginal malformations. J Pediatr Adolesc Gynecol. 2003;16(5):307–12. https://doi.org/10.1016/S1083-3188(03)00157-8.

Part II
Obstructive Uterine Malformation

Chapter 2
Mayer-Rokitansky-Küster-Hauser-Syndrome with Functional Endometrium

Sahra Steinmacher, Kristin Katharina Rall, and Sara Yvonne Brucker

Abstract The MRKH-syndrome is a congenital Müllerian duct anomaly and characterized by agenesis of the uterus and upper part of the vagina with normal ovarian function and female karyotype. Possible associated malformations include renal dysplasia, skeletal anomalies, or hearing defects. Its etiology is still unclear, ranging from a monogenic origin to a multifactorial or nongenetic etiology. Uterus remnants are seen in at least 50% of all patients.

Patients clinically present during adolescence with primary amenorrhea or refer to the impossibility of cohabitation. For initial diagnostics, transabdominal ultrasound can be performed to verify the absence of a uterus and presence of ovaries.

Magnetic resonance imaging serves as the gold standard for the confirmation of uterovaginal agenesis.

In the therapeutical management of vaginal agenesis, the nonsurgical and surgical techniques can be distinguished. Nonsurgical methods are based on a mechanical dilatation of the existing tissue. Surgical procedures comprise the use of autogenic transplants or the creation of a neovagina through dilatation with a traction device.

Besides surrogacy, uterus transplantation has additionally now arisen as an infertility treatment to provide motherhood.

Keywords MRKH syndrome · Uterovaginal agenesis

The Mayer-Rokitansky-Küster-Hauser (MRKH) syndrome is a congenital Müllerian duct anomaly. It is characterized by agenesis of the uterus and upper part of the vagina (2/3) with normal secondary sex characteristics and normal female karyotype.

The syndrome is divided into two subtypes: type I, which displays an isolated agenesis of uterus and vagina, and type II, which is associated with other malformations (MURCS association). Associated malformations include renal dysplasia such

S. Steinmacher (✉) · K. K. Rall · S. Y. Brucker
Department of Women's Health, Tuebingen University Hospital, Tuebingen, Germany
e-mail: sara.brucker@med.uni-tuebingen.de

L. Zhu et al. (eds.), *Diagnosis and Management of Female Obstructive Genital Malformations*, https://doi.org/10.1007/978-981-19-6759-7_2

as the existence of a horseshoe kidney, ectopia of kidneys or unilateral renal agenesis, skeletal and vertebral anomalies (scoliosis, fused vertebrae, Klippel-Feil syndrome), hearing defects, and rarely digital and cardiac anomalies.

MRKH syndrome occurs in about 1 of 4500 female live births [1–3]. MURCS association is less frequent than the isolated MRKH type I [4].

The etiology of MRKH remains unclear. A monogenic genetic origin is supported by the familial occurrence of MRKH syndrome and its associated malformations [5, 6]. On the other hand, reports of discordant twin pairs support rather a multifactorial or even nongenetic etiology [7–9].

Phenotypic presentation of the uterine aplasia may differ between the types of MRKH syndrome.

Type I often displays two aplastic uterine remnants on the pelvic wall. In type II, complete absence of one or both Müllerian ducts can be found and is often associated with ipsilateral kidney malformations.

Uterus remnants can be seen in 50% to almost 100% of all patients [10–12], whereas endometrium could be histologically detected in up to 50% of all surgically removed remnants [10, 13]. About 50% of these patients experience recurrent cyclic symptoms caused by the proliferation of the endometrium, endometriosis, or myomas [13–16], necessitating surgical or medical treatment [13]. Even hematometra can develop in the remnant cavity [17]. See Fig. 2.1 for a laparoscopic image of a bilateral prominent uterus remnant and Fig. 2.2 for the corresponding MRI image.

Moreover, uterus remnants in patients with Mayer-Rokitansky-Küster-Hauser (MRKH) syndrome were also found to have typical uterine tissue with a more basalis-like endometrium and significantly lower proliferation compared to healthy controls [10], possibly indicating a dysfunctional hormone receptor function that may play a role in the etiology of MRKHS.

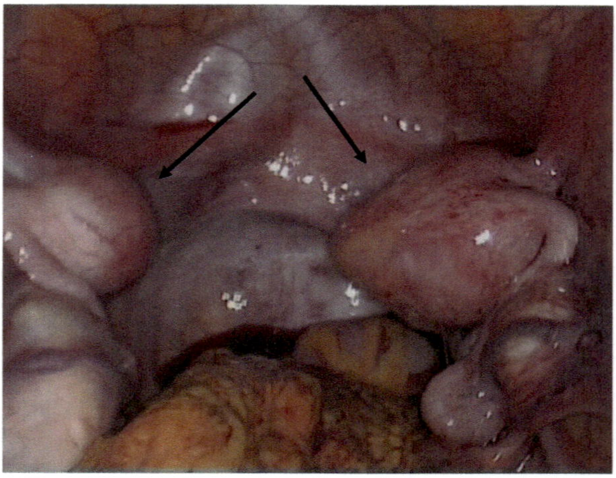

Fig. 2.1 Laparascopic image of a bilateral prominent uterus remnant

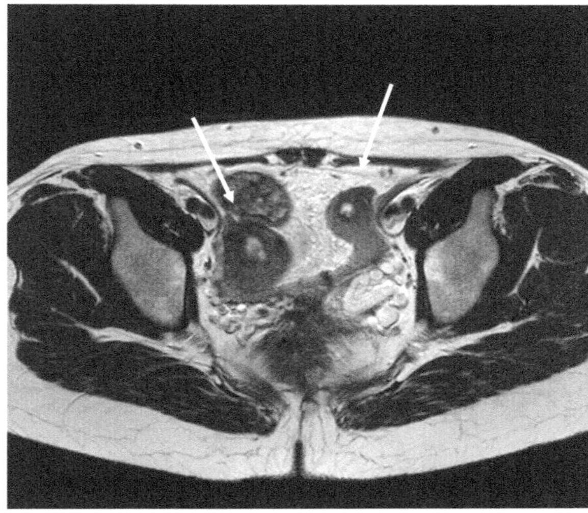

Fig. 2.2 Corresponding MRI image of the uterus remnant

2.1 Clinical Presentation and Diagnosis

Patients with MRKH syndrome present during adolescence with primary amenorrhea, defined by the absence of menstrual bleeding at the age of 16 after normal development of puberty and secondary sex characteristics, or due to the impossibility of cohabitation, and some report cyclic abdominal pain.

Patients with primary amenorrhea should be referred to a specialist in pediatric and adolescent gynecology. First, physical examination should be performed by inspection of the external genitalia and vagina. Here the patient's age should be taken into consideration, and vaginal examination should be avoided in prepubertal patients [18].

For initial diagnostics, transabdominal or rectal ultrasound can be performed to verify the absence of a uterus and presence of ovaries.

Magnetic resonance imaging serves as the gold standard for the confirmation of uterovaginal agenesis and can detect possible uterine remnants as well as existing endometrium. Moreover, atypically located ovaries can be detected and characterized, and possible malformations of the urinary tract, especially renal malformations, can be detected [12, 19]. A screening for possible extragenital malformations is not implemented yet in asymptomatic patients.

To confirm a normal female karyotype, chromosomal analysis is routinely performed.

Hormonal analysis confirms a normal hormonal function.

2.2 Differential Diagnosis

Other entities show phenotypic similarities to the features of MRKH. Complete androgen insensitivity syndrome (cAIS), as a 46 XY difference of sexual development (DSD), is an X-linked disorder affecting genetically males caused by mutations in the androgen receptor gene. cAIS is characterized by a normal female phenotype with normal breast development but aplasia of the upper vagina and uterus and sparse pubic and axillary hair.

17-Hydroxylase/17,20-lyase deficiency in 46,XY females displays mostly normal external genitalia, absence of uterus, and a shortened vagina.

To exclude potential differential diagnoses, chromosomal and hormonal analysis should be performed in order to distinguish MRKH syndrome from XY-DSD.

2.3 Management of Vaginal Agenesis

In the therapeutical management of vaginal agenesis, two types of procedure have to be distinguished: the nonsurgical and surgical techniques.

If suitable, the nonsurgical treatment to create a neovagina should be addressed primarily. It is recommended as the first-line treatment due to a relatively high success rate, its noninvasiveness, low costs, and low complication rates [20, 21].

Different treatment options should be discussed with the patient. Therefore, it should be pointed out that all therapeutic options to obtain a functional vagina require time and that consequent postoperative dilatation is also needed after surgery to guarantee an adequate long-term outcome, except after the creation of a sigmoid neovagina.

The patient should be counseled regarding the expectations for the treatment outcome and possible complications prior to any intervention. For a successful outcome, a high motivation level is mandatory.

Also, the option of no therapeutic intervention should be considered with the patient [22].

2.3.1 Nonsurgical Creation of a Neovagina

Nonsurgical methods are based on a mechanical dilatation of the existing tissue.

The most commonly used nonsurgical method is the progressive self-dilatation (Frank's method) [23]. Here vaginal dilators are manually placed with pressure on the vaginal apex for at least 20 min a day, progressively increasing in length and diameter. Treatment duration varies between weeks and in the majority of cases several months. This method should be applied when the vaginal length is already 2–4 cm before therapy and the yielded vaginal length is comparably short with an average length of 6.65 cm [24].

For this treatment option, a high compliance of the patient is needed, as an adequate treatment duration is necessary for a sufficient result and the therapy may be experienced as uncomfortable and painful [25]. Possible complications include accidental urethral dilatation, vaginal shrinkage, or prolapse [26].

2.3.2 Surgical Creation of a Neovagina

For surgical creation of a neovagina, various techniques are applied.

1. *Abbe-McIndoe Technique (Using Autogenic Transplants)*
   Here, a surgical tunneling of a space between the rectum and the bladder to the Douglas pouch is created. A vaginal dummy is placed covered with an autogenic skin graft into the space and is removed after a few days. Postoperative frequent vaginal dilatation has to be performed. Advantages of this technique are the nonabdominal access and the comparably simple surgical technique [25, 26]. Possible disadvantages include a rejection of the transplant, secondary stenosis, and a risk of fistula. In comparison to other surgical methods, the McIndoe technique has the highest rate of infections and reoperations [26].
2. *Davydov Vaginoplasty (Using Autogenic Transplants)*
   The laparoscopically performed Davydov technique combines a vesicorectal tunneling with the transplantation of autogenic tissue. After dissection of the vesicorectal space, the peritoneum of the Douglas pouch is mobilized and formed to provide the neovagina [27]. Potential complications include the risk of intestinal or bladder injury, vaginal prolapse, and postoperative infections. Further reported disadvantages are vaginal stenosis or vaginal granulation tissue [27].
3. *Skin Flap Vaginoplasty (Using Autogenic Transplants)*
   For neovagina creation, full skin transplants can be applied by using flaps originating from the vulvoperineal, gluteal, or gracilis region. Postoperative shrinkage of the transplant is considerably low, but this technique displays an increased risk of scarring, dehiscence, or intravaginal hair growth [27]. For the Williams vulvovaginoplasty, the labia majora are sutured into a perineal pouch, thus forming a neovagina [28].
4. *Intestinal Vaginoplasty (Using Autogenic Transplants)*
   This technique involves a neovaginal creation by grafting a segment of sigmoid. Primarily, the vesicorectal space is tunneled and the sigmoid transplant is then inserted and fixed at the introitus.

   Despite the high success rates, injury or bleeding of the rectum and the risk of re-laparotomy are reported as intraoperative complications. Extended neovaginal shrinkage, anastomosis insufficiency, and extended vaginal discharge can occur postoperatively [29]. Furthermore, prolapse of the neovagina, colitis ulcerosa, and development of adenocarcinoma are reported [26].
5. *Wharton-Sheares-George Vaginoplasty (Method Without Transplants)*
   For a neovagina creation using the Wharton-Sheares-George method, the vesicorectal space is dissected without the usage of a transplant. A vaginal

dummy is inserted daily for 3 months after a previous probing of the obliterated Müllerian ducts [30]. Patients receiving this technique show a persistent adequate vaginal length, low occurrence of contractions, and a physiological epithelial lining [31]. In order to avoid a subsequent stenosis, lifelong dilatation is necessary. This method also carries the risk of rectoceles and cystoceles [32].

6. *Modified Vecchietti Technique*

   The modified Vecchietti technique combines surgical and nonsurgical methods [33]. Two threads attached to a plastic olive are brought through the vaginal dimple into the abdominal cavity under laparoscopic view, nowadays without the need for abdominovaginal dissection of the vesicorectal space. The creation of a neovagina is then performed through dilatation with a traction device attached to the abdominal wall. Via continuous pressure on the vaginal dimple, a neovagina is created within 4–5 days [34]. In 1992, the laparoscopic route had been established and continuously optimized through modifications avoiding an open abdominal approach [33, 35].

   Advantages of this technique include the lack of need of a transplant, a physiological epithelial lining with all functions usually characterizing the normal vagina, and is even possible when a pelvic kidney is present [36]. The method offers a minimally traumatic procedure with a very low number of long-term complications [37].

2.4 Infertility Treatment and Uterus Transplantation

Patients with MRKH syndrome suffer from absolute uterine factor infertility, comprising women with complete anatomical absence or presence of a nonfunctioning uterus.

As motherhood options serve adoption or gestational surrogacy, in vitro fertilization is performed first with oocytes from the patient and her partner's sperm. The embryo is then transferred to the gestational surrogate carrier [18].

Uterus transplantation has additionally now arisen as an infertility treatment to provide genetic, gestational, and legal motherhood. The first live birth after uterus transplantation took place in 2014 in Gothenburg, Sweden [38].

As the uterus transplantation is performed with a living donor in most countries, a rigid preoperative selection including physical examinations with immunological testing and psychological assessments is performed to ensure safety of donor and recipient and thus the success of the uterus transplantation [39–41].

In order to shorten the time of immune suppression to the only necessary level, explantation of the uterus is performed after the completion of family planning.

2.5 Conclusion

Vaginal and uterine aplasia due to MRKH syndrome is the second most common cause for primary amenorrhea. Patients usually present with asymptomatic primary amenorrhea between 15 and 17 years of age only. Nevertheless, from our experience, more than half of the patients suffer from cyclic lower abdominal pain due to Mittelschmerz or existing endometrium inside the uterine rudiments, and even endometriosis and myomas have been described.

Associated malformations of the kidneys and lower urinary tract as well as other organs should be kept in mind.

Nonsurgical and different surgical methods for the creation of a neovagina have been described, and the method of choice is dependent on the patient's wish and history and on the experience of the gynecologist. Symptomatic uterine rudiments can be removed if necessary.

Motherhood can be possible with adoption, surrogacy, or uterus transplantation in strictly selected patients.

References

1. Varner RE, Younger JB, Blackwell RE. Mullerian dysgenesis. J Reprod Med. 1985;30(6):443–50.
2. Aittomaki K, Eroila H, Kajanoja P. A population-based study of the incidence of Mullerian aplasia in Finland. Fertil Steril. 2001;76(3):624–5.
3. Folch M, Pigem I, Konje JC. Mullerian agenesis: etiology, diagnosis, and management. Obstet Gynecol Surv. 2000;55(10):644–9.
4. Strubbe EH, et al. The Mayer-Rokitansky-Kuster-Hauser (MRKH) syndrome without and with associated features: two separate entities? Clin Dysmorphol. 1994;3(3):192–9.
5. Herlin M, Hojland AT, Petersen MB. Familial occurrence of Mayer-Rokitansky-Kuster-Hauser syndrome: a case report and review of the literature. Am J Med Genet A. 2014;164A(9):2276–86.
6. Williams LS, et al. Genetic analysis of Mayer-Rokitansky-Kuster-Hauser syndrome in a large cohort of families. Fertil Steril. 2017;108(1):145–51 e2.
7. Regenstein AC, Berkeley AS. Discordance of Mullerian agenesis in monozygotic twins. *A case report*. J Reprod Med. 1991;36(5):396–7.
8. Duru UA, Laufer MR. Discordance in Mayer-von Rokitansky-Kuster-Hauser syndrome noted in monozygotic twins. J Pediatr Adolesc Gynecol. 2009;22(4):e73–5.
9. Milsom SR, et al. Discordant Mayer-Rokitansky-Kuster-Hauser (MRKH) syndrome in identical twins – a case report and implications for reproduction in MRKH women. Gynecol Endocrinol. 2015;31(9):684–7.
10. Rall K, et al. Uterine rudiments in patients with Mayer-Rokitansky-Kuster-Hauser syndrome consist of typical uterine tissue types with predominantly basalis-like endometrium. Fertil Steril. 2013;99(5):1392–9.
11. Oppelt PG, et al. Malformations in a cohort of 284 women with Mayer-Rokitansky-Kuster-Hauser syndrome (MRKH). Reprod Biol Endocrinol. 2012;10:57.

12. Preibsch H, et al. Clinical value of magnetic resonance imaging in patients with Mayer-Rokitansky-Kuster-Hauser (MRKH) syndrome: diagnosis of associated malformations, uterine rudiments and intrauterine endometrium. Eur Radiol. 2014;24(7):1621–7.
13. Marsh CA, et al. Uterine remnants and pelvic pain in females with Mayer-Rokitansky-Kuster-Hauser syndrome. J Pediatr Adolesc Gynecol. 2013;26(3):199–202.
14. Fedele L, et al. Laparoscopic findings and pelvic anatomy in Mayer-Rokitansky-Kuster-Hauser syndrome. Obstet Gynecol. 2007;109(5):1111–5.
15. Deligeoroglou E, et al. Development of leiomyomas on the uterine remnants of two women with Mayer-Rokitansky-Kuster-Hauser syndrome. Fertil Steril. 2004;81(5):1385–7.
16. Papa G, et al. Case report and surgical solution for a voluminous uterine leiomyoma in a woman with complicated Mayer-Rokitansky-Kuster-Hauser syndrome. Fertil Steril. 2008;90(5):2014 e5-6.
17. Howard LA, Mancuso AC, Ryan GL. Mullerian aplasia with severe hematometra: a case report of diagnosis and management in a low resource setting. J Pediatr Adolesc Gynecol. 2019;32(2):189–92.
18. Herlin MK, Petersen MB, Brannstrom M. Mayer-Rokitansky-Kuster-Hauser (MRKH) syndrome: a comprehensive update. Orphanet J Rare Dis. 2020;15(1):214.
19. Lermann J, et al. Comparison of different diagnostic procedures for the staging of malformations associated with Mayer-Rokitansky-Kuster-Hauser syndrome. Fertil Steril. 2011;96(1):156–9.
20. Committee on Adolescent Health Care. ACOG Committee Opinion No. 728: Mullerian agenesis: diagnosis, management, and treatment. Obstet Gynecol. 2018;131(1):e35–42.
21. American College of Obstetrics and Gynecology Committee on Adolescent Health Care. ACOG Committee Opinion. Number 274, July 2002. Nonsurgical diagnosis and management of vaginal agenesis. Int J Gynaecol Obstet. 2002;79(2):167–70.
22. Dear J, et al. Sexual experience before treatment for vaginal agenesis: a retrospective review of 137 women. J Pediatr Adolesc Gynecol. 2019;32(3):300–4.
23. Williams B. Formation of an artificial vagina by Frank's method. J Obstet Gynaecol Br Emp. 1957;64(2):241–2.
24. McQuillan SK, Grover SR. Dilation and surgical management in vaginal agenesis: a systematic review. Int Urogynecol J. 2014;25(3):299–311.
25. Nakhal RS, Creighton SM. Management of vaginal agenesis. J Pediatr Adolesc Gynecol. 2012;25(6):352–7.
26. Callens N, et al. An update on surgical and non-surgical treatments for vaginal hypoplasia. Hum Reprod Update. 2014;20(5):775–801.
27. Davydov SN, Zhvitiashvili OD. Formation of vagina (colpopoiesis) from peritoneum of Douglas pouch. Acta Chir Plast. 1974;16(1):35–41.
28. Williams EA. Congenital absence of the vagina: a simple operation for its relief. J Obstet Gynaecol Br Commonw. 1964;71:511–2.
29. Carrard C, et al. Sexuality after sigmoid vaginoplasty in patients with Mayer-Rokitansky-Kuster-Hauser syndrome. Fertil Steril. 2012;97(3):691–6.
30. Schatz T, Huber J, Wenzl R. Creation of a neovagina according to Wharton-Sheares-George in patients with Mayer-Rokitansky-Kuster-Hauser syndrome. Fertil Steril. 2005;83(2):437–41.
31. Walch K, et al. Functional and anatomic results after creation of a neovagina according to Wharton-Sheares-George in patients with Mayer-Rokitansky-Kuster-Hauser syndrome-long-term follow-up. Fertil Steril. 2011;96(2):492–97 e1.
32. Kuhn A, et al. Prolapse and sexual function 8 years after neovagina according to shears: a study of 43 cases with Mayer-von Rokitansky-Kuster-Hauser syndrome. Int Urogynecol J. 2013;24(6):1047–52.
33. Brucker SY, et al. Neovagina creation in vaginal agenesis: development of a new laparoscopic Vecchietti-based procedure and optimized instruments in a prospective comparative interventional study in 101 patients. Fertil Steril. 2008;90(5):1940–52.
34. Vecchietti G. Creation of an artificial vagina in Rokitansky-Kuster-Hauser syndrome. Attual Ostet Ginecol. 1965;11(2):131–47.

35. Gauwerky JF, Wallwiener D, Bastert G. An endoscopically assisted technique for construction of a neovagina. Arch Gynecol Obstet. 1992;252(2):59–63.
36. Fedele L, et al. Neovaginal mucosa after Vecchietti's laparoscopic operation for Rokitansky syndrome: structural and ultrastructural study. Am J Obstet Gynecol. 2006;195(1):56–61.
37. Rall K, et al. Laparoscopically assisted neovaginoplasty in vaginal agenesis: a long-term outcome study in 240 patients. J Pediatr Adolesc Gynecol. 2014;27(6):379–85.
38. Brannstrom M, et al. Livebirth after uterus transplantation. Lancet. 2015;385(9968):607–16.
39. Taran FA, et al. Screening and evaluation of potential recipients and donors for living donor uterus transplantation: results from a single-center observational study. Fertil Steril. 2019;111(1):186–93.
40. Johannesson L, et al. Living uterus donation and transplantation: experience of interest and screening in a single center in the United States. Am J Obstet Gynecol. 2018;218(3):331 e1–7.
41. Brucker SY, et al. Living-donor uterus transplantation: pre-, intra-, and postoperative parameters relevant to surgical success, pregnancy, and obstetrics with live births. J Clin Med. 2020;9(8):2485.

Chapter 3
Unicornuate Uterus Complicated with Rudimentary Horn Uterus with Functional Endometrium

Xinmiao Bao, Na Chen, and Lan Zhu

Abstract The unicornuate uterus is a rare congenital uterine anomaly. Most unicornuate uteri present with contralateral rudimentary horn uterus with functional endometrium. Patients with functional rudimentary horn uterus usually present with dysmenorrhea and may complicate with malformation of fallopian tube and urinary system. Transvaginal pelvic ultrasound is the first-line diagnostic method, and hysteroscopic-united laparoscopic examination is the gold standard for diagnosis. Rudimentary horn uterus and the ipsilateral fallopian tube resection should be performed once diagnosed to relieve symptoms and to prevent rudimentary horn uterus pregnancy. Postoperative management should focus on monitoring adverse obstetrics outcomes such as recurrent pregnancy loss, intrauterine growth restriction, and preterm delivery.

Keywords Unicornuate uterus · Rudimentary horn uterus · Functional endometrium · Uterus anomaly · Congenital malformation

The unicornuate uterus is a rare congenital uterine anomaly with a prevalence of 1/5400 [1]. It is caused by abnormal or failed development of one Mullerian duct. In 1988, the American Fertility Society (AFS) proposed a classification system for Mullerian anomalies, classifying unicornuate uterus as class II. Based on the anatomical relationship between the unicornuate uterus and complicated rudimentary uterus, class II is further divided into (1) class IIa: the rudimentary horn cavity communicates with the uterus, (2) class IIb: the rudimentary horn cavity does not communicate with the uterus, (3) class IIc: the rudimentary horn does not have a cavity, and (4) class IId: no horn [2]. The European Society of Human Reproduction and Embryology (ESHRE) and the European Society of

X. Bao (✉) · N. Chen · L. Zhu
National Clinical Research Center for Obstetric and Gynecologic Diseases, Department of Obstetrics and Gynecology, State Key Laboratory of Complex Severe and Rare Diseases, Peking Union Medical College Hospital, Peking Union Medical College and Chinese Academy of Medical Sciences, Beijing, China
e-mail: xinmiao.bao@berkeley.edu

L. Zhu et al. (eds.), *Diagnosis and Management of Female Obstructive Genital Malformations*, https://doi.org/10.1007/978-981-19-6759-7_3

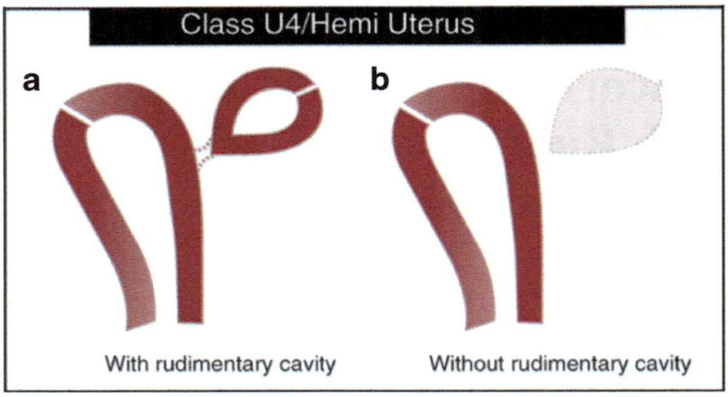

Fig. 3.1 ESHRE/ESGE classification. (From [3])

Gynaecological Endoscopy (ESGE) established another classification of uterine anomalies, with unicornuate uterus being class U4, which is further divided into two subclasses depending on the presence or not of a functional rudimentary cavity [3]: (1) class U4a: hemi uterus with a rudimentary cavity (communicating or not horn). (2) class U4b: hemi uterus without rudimentary cavity (horn without cavity/no horn) (Fig. 3.1). Contralateral rudimentary uterine exists in about 74%–90% of the unicornuate uterus [4]. This chapter mainly discusses the unicornuate uterus with functional rudimentary horn.

3.1 Clinical Manifestation

Patients can be asymptomatic due to the lack of functional endometrium, considering the menstrual outflow is non-obstructed. However, patients with noncommunicating rudimentary horn uterus with functional endometrium can present with progressively aggravated dysmenorrhea. Dysmenorrhea and lower abdominal pain can also be caused by endometriosis or chronic pelvic inflammatory disease due to retrograde menstruation. In addition, dysplasia in the fimbriated end of the fallopian tube and urological abnormalities are often complicated on the side unilateral to the rudimentary horn uterus. The incidence of renal malformations can be as high as 40%, mainly present in horseshoe kidney, double collecting system, and ectopic kidney [5]. Among these, renal agenesis is the most frequently associated urinary tract abnormality [6].

3.2 Signs

Rudimentary horn uterus is difficult to detect by bimanual examination. Rudimentary horn uterus with hematometra should be considered in addition to adenomyosis or ovarian tumor if a mass closely proximate to the uterus is palpable in a patient with dysmenorrhea.

3.3 Complications

Functional endometrial tissue within the rudimentary horn may cause endometriosis, pelvic adhesion, and other complications [7], especially in the noncommunicating rudimentary uterus, where retrograde menstruation is more prominent. Hence, the prevalence of complicating any type of endometriosis (superficial, ovarian, or deep) in patients with functional rudimentary uterus is relatively high. This may be one of the main causes of their adverse reproductive outcomes such as infertility and ectopic pregnancy [8].

3.4 Diagnosis

3.4.1 Examination

Main diagnostic examinations include pelvic ultrasound, magnetic resonance imaging (MRI), hysterosalpingography (HSG), hysteroscopy, and laparoscopy:

1. 2D ultrasound: Transvaginal (or transrectal for patients who had no sexual activity) pelvic ultrasound is the first-line diagnostic method; two-dimensional ultrasound of the unicornuate uterus shows [9] (1) asymmetrical uterine configuration with the cervix on a different plane when viewing on the transverse section, (2) the endometrium on the fundus only show unicornuate horn, (3) lack of continuity between the uterus and fallopian tube, (4) possible absence of ipsilateral kidney and ovary, and (5) rudimentary horn uterus can be detected as a solid structure with or without endometrium on one side.
2. Pelvic MRI: The unicornuate uterus being narrow and deviated to one side of the pelvis. Fat-suppressed T2W1 can demonstrate the three layers of the uterus. For class U4a, a small cavity with a high signal intensity endometrial-like structure can be detected, and a larger rudimentary cavity can even show a complete junction zone. Anatomic features and relationships between the unicornuate uterus and rudimentary horn can be seen on thin coronal sections. A dilated fluid-filled structure, which appears to be hyperintense on T1W1, might be detected in class U4a anomaly (Fig. 3.2).
3. Hysterosalpingography (HSG): Irregularity of uterine contour and unilateral scarring of the cavity. Only one side of the fallopian tube communicates with the uterus (Fig. 3.3). The rudimentary horn uterus can be shown to connect to the leaf-shaped unicornuate uterus with a thin band. However, many rudimentary uteri do not communicate with the unicornuate uterus. Therefore, the diagnostic value of HSG in the rudimentary uterus is limited.
4. Hysteroscopic-united laparoscopic examination: The gold standard of unicornuate uterus anomaly. Only one oviduct inlet can be visualized under hysteroscopy (Fig. 3.4). Together with laparoscopy, both the uterus' internal morphology and

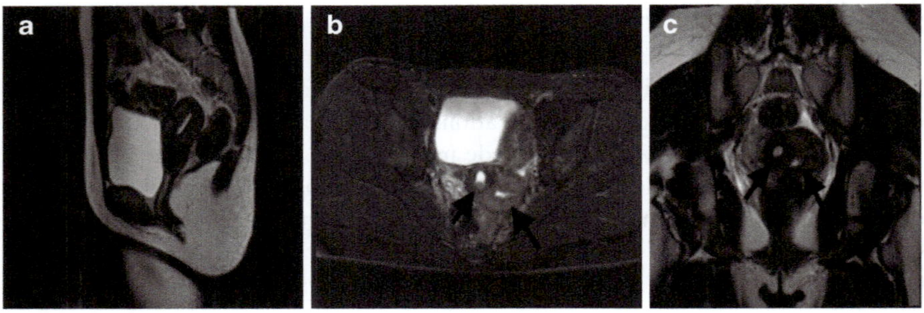

Fig. 3.2 Pelvic magnetic resonance imaging of a patient with unicornuate uterus with rudimentary horn. (**a**) Sagittal plane. (**b**) Fat-suppressed T2WI in cross-sectioned plane. (**c**) Thin coronal section, showing left unicornuate uterus (black long arrow) and right rudimentary horn uterus (black short arrow)

Fig. 3.3 HSG of unicornuate uterus shows filling of the dominant right unicornuate horn (white arrow) and right fallopian tube (white arrowhead). No contrast is seen in the expected location of the left horn. [10]

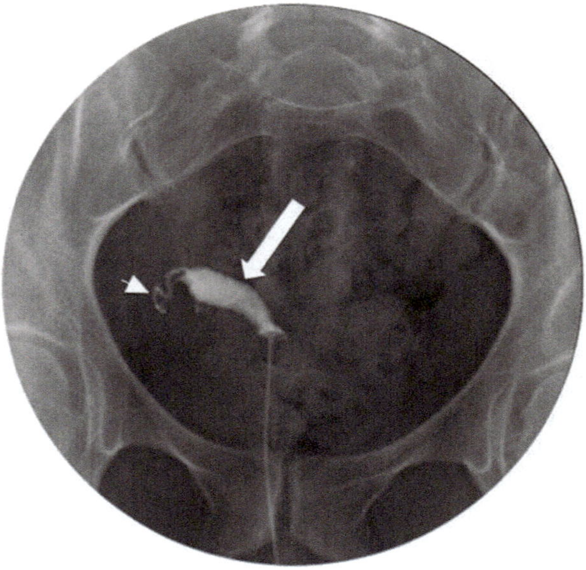

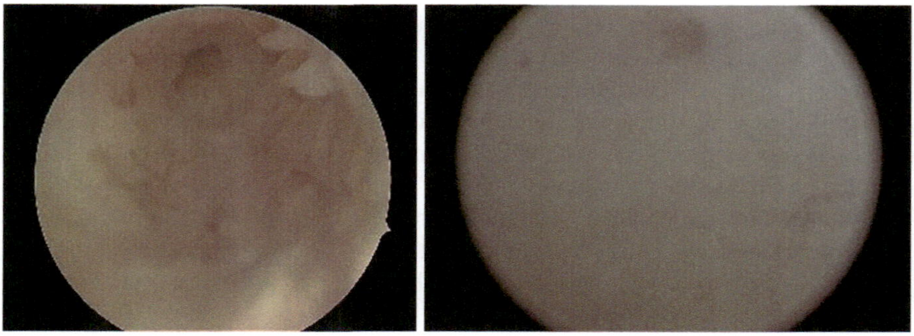

Fig. 3.4 Only one oviduct inlet can be seen under hysteroscopy

external outline can be directly visualized, helping the correct typing of the anomaly. Furthermore, physicians can simultaneously perform rudimentary horn resection, achieving diagnosis and treatment at the same time.

3.4.2 *Differential Diagnosis*

1. Bicornuate uterus: Needs to be differentiated from the unicornuate uterus with communicating rudimentary horn. Coronal MRI images of the bicornuate uterus usually reveal Y-shape uterine cavity, and the two cavities fuse above the internal cervical os. The distance between the two horns is generally >4 cm, the angle >105°, and the fundal indent depth is 2 ~ 3 cm. While unicornuate uterus is smaller in volume and has a narrow lower uterine cavity, the endometrium shows a long T2 signal on MRI in a "banana-shaped" structure on one side of the pelvis. The rudimentary horn is shown as a round structure with isointense T1 and hypointensity T2 signals. The center can be nonhomogeneous hyperintensity when hematometra is present.
2. Didelphys uterus: Two uteri exist independently, resulting in two separate endometrial cavities and two cervices. Each uterus has an endometrium, junction zone, and muscular layer. Most patients are complicated with a transverse vaginal septum.
3. Accessory-cavitated uterine mass (ACUM): Present as a round cystic mass lined by the endometrium, with blood products contained, usually adjacent to the normal-shaped uterine cavity at the level of the round ligament. The radiological presentation is similar to that of a noncommunicating rudimentary horn uterus. However, the uterine configuration unicornuate uterus with functional rudimentary horn is asymmetric with only one side of the fallopian tube connected to the uterus, while ACUM has normal uterine and fallopian tube anatomy. The hysteroscopic-united laparoscopic examination can facilitate differentiation.

3.5 Treatment

The preferred standard treatment is the surgical resection of the rudimentary uterine horn. The removal of functional noncommunicating rudimentary horn uterus can relieve pain and prevent endometriosis caused by retrograde menstrual flow [11]. Although communicating rudimentary horn uterus often does not present with dysmenorrhea, there is still a risk of rudimentary horn pregnancy leading to life--threatening uterine rupture. Therefore, rudimentary horn uterus resection should be performed once diagnosed. Either laparoscopy or laparotomy is preferred, but the laparoscopic removal of a rudimentary horn is more common (Fig. 3.5). Meanwhile, the fallopian tube ipsilateral to the rudimentary horn uterus should also be removed to prevent an ectopic tubal pregnancy.

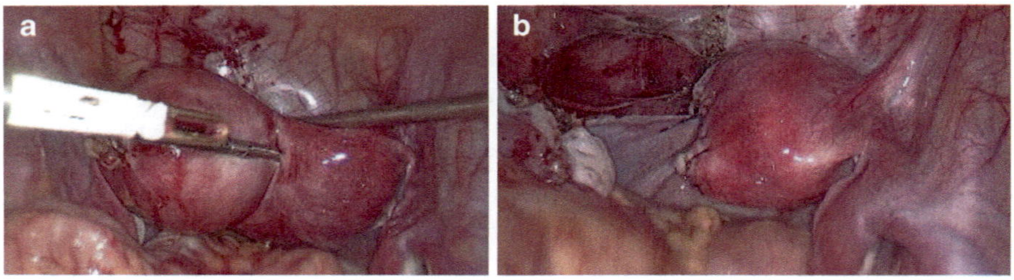

Fig. 3.5 Laparoscopic view of the unicornuate uterus in situ. (**a**) Two uterine bodies can be seen before surgery. (**b**) After surgery

Intraoperatively, light-guided hysteroscopy can help locate the junction plane between the unicornuate and rudimentary uterus, followed by the separation of the two uteri along the plane. When excising the noncommunicating rudimentary uterus, complete removal of endometrium should be guaranteed, while the complete resection of rudimentary horn myometrium is not strictly required. Pay great attention not to damage the unicornuate uterus, especially when the attachment in between is tight and extensive [12]. The excised rudimentary horn uterus can be pulled out by enlarging the suprapubic TROCAR incision or transvaginally. Lastly, the unicornuate uterus is sutured layer by layer.

3.6 Postoperative Management and Reproductive Outcome

Postoperative medication is not regularly used if no endometriosis is complicated. Complications such as endometriosis can be treated accordingly.

For patients who have fertility needs post-surgery, close monitoring during the second and third trimesters is recommended due to the relative decrease in the mass of uterine myometrium. Recurrent pregnancy loss, intrauterine growth restriction, and preterm delivery should be alerted.

In addition, be cautious with a rare condition—rudimentary horn uterine pregnancy. A functional rudimentary horn uterus can be fertilized because it has periodic menstruation. Pregnancies in rudimentary horns can occur following transperitoneal migration of sperm or zygote. While communicating rudimentary horn uterus has a higher pregnancy rate due to richer blood flow, thicker myometrium results in longer gestational weeks than the noncommunicating rudimentary uterus. Pregnancy in a noncommunicating rudimentary horn is extremely rare and is associated with maternal mortality. Rupture mainly occurs in the second trimester leading to severe intra-abdominal bleeding and high maternal mortality. Hence, the rudimentary horn uterus and the ipsilateral fallopian tube should be surgically removed immediately upon diagnosis. In rare cases, noncommunicating rudimentary horn uterus pregnancy can reach term, requiring cesarean section. Even more rarely, simultaneous pregnancy involving the unicornuate uterus and rudimentary horn uterus has been reported.

References

1. Letterie GS. Management of congenital uterine abnormalities. Reprod Biomed Online. 2011;23(1):40–52.
2. The American Fertility Society classifications of adnexal adhesions, distal tubal occlusion, tubal occlusion secondary to tubal ligation, tubal pregnancies, Müllerian anomalies and intrauterine adhesions. Fertil Steril. 1988;49(6):944–55.
3. Grimbizis GF, Gordts S, Di Spiezio SA, et al. The ESHRE/ESGE consensus on the classification of female genital tract congenital anomalies. Hum Reprod. 2013;28(8):2032–44.
4. Zhang Y, Liu S, Zhang X, et al. Laparoscopic metroplasty for unicornuate uterus with a functional noncommunicating rudimentary horn. Int J Gynaecol Obstet. 2020;149(1):31–6.
5. Fedele L, Bianchi S, Agnoli B, et al. Urinary tract anomalies associated with unicornuate uterus. J Urol. 1996;155(3):847–8.
6. Buttram VC Jr, Gibbons WE. Müllerian anomalies: a proposed classification. (An analysis of 144 cases). Fertil Steril. 1979;32(1):40–6.
7. Tian W, Chen N, Liang Z, et al. Clinical features and management of endometriosis among patients with MRKH and functional uterine remnants. Gynecol Obstet Invest. 2021;86(6):518–24.
8. Piriyev E, Römer T. Coincidence of uterine malformations and endometriosis: a clinically relevant problem? Arch Gynecol Obstet. 2020;302(5):1237–41.
9. Khati NJ, Frazier AA, Brindle KA. The unicornuate uterus and its variants: clinical presentation, imaging findings, and associated complications. J Ultrasound Med. 2012;31(2):319–31.
10. Dove CK, Harvey SM, Spalluto LB. Reprinted from "Sonographic findings of early pregnancy in the rudimentary horn of a unicornuate uterus: a two case report". Clin Imaging. 2018;47:25–9. Copyright (2018), with permission from Elsevier
11. Faller E, Baldauf JJ, Becmeur F, et al. Laparoscopic management of a rudimentary uterine horn. J Minim Invasive Gynecol. 2018;25(5):769–70.
12. Yen CF, Hsin-Yu Pai A, Lo A, et al. Laparoscopic metroplasty: reconstructive surgery for unicornuate uterus with noncommunicating, functional uterine horn. Fertil Steril. 2020;114(5):1119–21.

Chapter 4
Robert's Uterus

Xiaochuan Li, Shan Deng, and Lan Zhu

Abstract Robert's uterus is a rare subtype of the septate uterus by the Müllerian malformations classification, which is described as "asymmetric septate uterus." In this chapter, we discuss the symptoms and diagnosis of Robert's uterus. In addition, the treatments and prognoses will also be introduced briefly.

Keywords Robert's uterus · Asymmetric septate uterus

Robert's uterus was named after being first reported by Dr. Robert in 1970 [1]. It is described as "asymmetric septate uterus," and less than 100 cases have been reported in the literature until now. Robert's uterus is considered a subtype of the septate uterus by the Müllerian malformations classification published by the American Society for Reproductive Medicine (ASRM) [2] and the European Society of Human Reproduction and Embryology (ESHRE) & the European Society of Gynecologic Endoscopy (ESGE). However, unlike the classical septate uterus, the septum in Robert's uterus is biased to one side of the uterine cavity, completely sealing the lateral uterine cavity without communicating with the cervix, vagina, and contralateral uterine cavity, as shown in Fig. 4.1. It has been reported that the right blind cavity is more common in Robert's uterus, which is possibly attributed to the left Müllerian tube developing slightly earlier than the right side.

X. Li · S. Deng · L. Zhu (✉)
Department of Obstetrics and Gynecology, Peking Union Medical College Hospital, Peking Union Medical College, Beijing, China

L. Zhu et al. (eds.), *Diagnosis and Management of Female Obstructive Genital Malformations*, https://doi.org/10.1007/978-981-19-6759-7_4

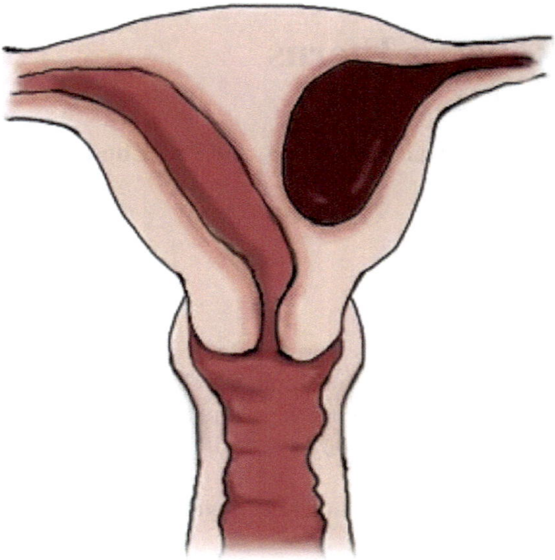

Fig. 4.1 Schematic diagram of Robert's uterus

4.1 Symptoms

Due to the blind cavity with functional endometrium in Robert's uterus, almost all the patients may present obstructive symptoms, especially in adolescent girls shortly after menarche. According to the size of the blind cavity, the function of the fallopian tube, and the duration of the course, primary dysmenorrhea or progressive aggravating dysmenorrhea may be seen in patients. Endometriosis or infertility may also be present as secondary diseases.

When the intrauterine septum is in the upper half of the uterus, the blind cavity is very small and the clinical symptoms may be mild; when the septum ends at the lower, the blind cavity is large with massive blood accumulation and severe dysmenorrhea [3].

4.2 Signs

Physical examination findings include a single uterus with one normal cervix but a wide fundus. The uterine tenderness can be found. As the disease progresses, pelvic or ovarian endometriosis can develop, presenting with an adnexal mass or tender rectovaginal nodules.

4.3 Complications and Pregnancy Outcomes

Due to the abnormal cavity of the uterus, most patients with Robert's uterus suffer from infertility, secondary hemosalpinx, and pelvic and ovarian endometriosis. There have also been reports of early pregnancy in the blind cavity [4].

4.4 Diagnosis

4.4.1 Diagnostic Criteria

The key point of the diagnosis is the "closed septum" communicating with the fallopian tube. The appearance of the uterus can be normal, wide in the fundus, or asymmetrical enlargement in the uterine corpus. Hysteroscopy or uterosalpingogram showed a uterus with an oblique septum connected with the tubal opening. Hysteroscopy combined with uterine laparoscopy is the gold standard for the diagnosis of Robert's uterus.

Some resachers [5] further divided Robert's uterus into three types: (1) large blind cavity with acute abdominal pain; (2) non-functional blind cavity with repeated abortion; and (3) small blind cavity with a small amount of blood accumulation. The above phenotype is closely related to the functional amount of the endometrium in the blind cavity and the function of the fallopian tube. It is important to identify the combined signs such as blood accumulation in the tube, which may cause greater difficulty in the diagnosis.

4.4.2 Diagnostic Method

1. Ultrasound: Compared with two-dimensional ultrasound, three-dimensional ultrasound provides a better coronal section of the uterus, the intrauterine septum, and the shape of the uterine floor.
2. Uterine salpingography (HSG)

   As HSG could not assess the whole uterine appearance, it is not sufficient for the diagnosis of Robert's uterus alone. The HSG performance in Robert's uterus is the same as the unicornuate uterus or type II residual uterine horn.
3. Magnetic resonance imaging (MRI)

   As a rare disease, the patient with a suspected diagnosis should receive an MRI scan, especially for the preoperative evaluation. Two uterine cavities divided by an asymmetric septum can be found (Fig. 4.2). Hematometra of the uterine cavity and fallopian tube may be present as a result of the obstruction in the uterine cavity and cervical canal.
4. Hysteroscopy and laparoscopy

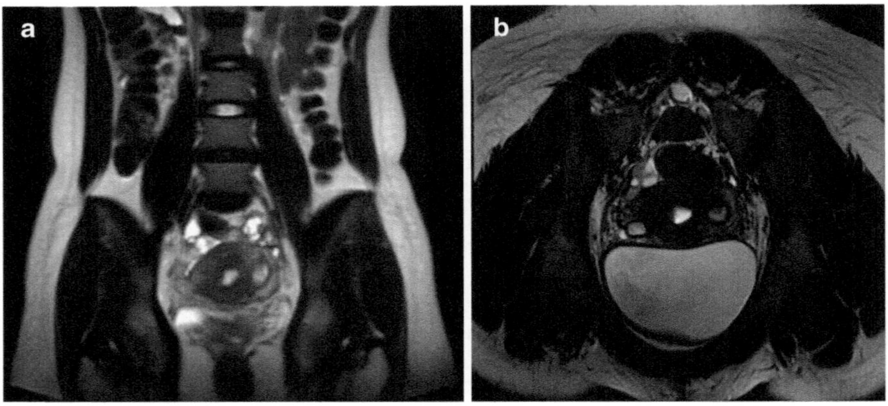

Fig. 4.2 MRI scan of Robert's uterus (MRI scan in coronal (**a**) and axial (**b**) planes)

Laparoscopic examination showed a roughly normal uterine appearance. Hematometra in the blind cavity may lead to swelling at the uterine horn. It is different from the bicornuate uterus because hysteroscopy revealed a tubular cavity similar to the unicornuate uterus, with only a unilateral tubal opening.

4.4.3 Differential Diagnosis

1. Accessory and cavitated uterine mass (ACUM): It is an extremely rare disease characterized by a cavitated mass located between the round ligament and the uterus, with an endometrial cavity filled with accumulated blood. From the pathogenesis, ACUM is considered to be the abnormal development of the Müllerian tube in the round ligament area or related to the lead band dysfunction, and its blind cavity is not connected to the fallopian tube. However, Robert's uterus is a special type of uterine septum, and its blind cavity is actually part of the uterine cavity. Robert's uterus with a larger blind cavity has a locally convex fundus, which may be similar to ACUM in appearance. However, hysteroscopy of ACUM patients shows bilateral normal tubal opening, which can be distinguished from Robert's uterus.
2. Unicornuate uterus combined with type II rudimentary horn: It is a combination of one functional rudimentary horn on one side and the unicornuate on the other side. But Robert's uterus has a single uterine body with a normal appearance.
3. Oblique vaginal septum syndrome: The oblique septum is in the vagina below the cervix. The oblique septum in Robert's uterus is in the uterine cavity.
4. Juvenile cystic adenomyoma (JCA): It is also very rare. Takeuchi et al. [6] proposed the diagnostic criteria for juvenile cystic adenomyosis in 2010 as follows: (1) $\leq$30 years old; (2) the cyst $\geq$1 cm and independent from the uterine cavity, with hyperplasia of smooth muscle; and (3) severe dysmenorrhea. The clinical

symptoms of JCA can be similar to those of Robert's uterus, but its cystic lesions are located in the myometrium, with ectopic endometrium. Uterine salpingography (HSG) examination showed normal uterine cavity morphology; imaging suggested a cyst in the myometrium, with chocolate-like fluid in the pathological cavity and smooth muscle tissue covered.

4.5 Treatment

Surgery is the only effective way to treat Robert's uterus. Previous literature reported transabdominal or laparoscopic hemihysterectomy [7] and endometrial ablation of the blind cavity. In recent years, more hysteroscopic surgeries have been reported, such as the hysteroscopic incision of the uterine oblique septum. It removes the obstruction and restores the uterine cavity. In addition, laparoscopic treatment of pelvic or ovarian endometriosis is also performed.

4.6 Postoperative Management and Prognosis

The key point of postoperative management includes the prevention of intrauterine adhesions, follow-up menstrual conditions, and improve fertility. It is recommended to place a uterine cavity balloon or other barrier anti-adhesive agent to prevent intrauterine adhesions. If necessary, a repeat hysteroscopy is performed to evaluate the recovery of the uterine cavity. Xia enlan et al. [8] reported 11 cases of Robert's uterus in China, which is the biggest population in the world. Patients at diagnosis were 15–19 years, with a history of dysmenorrhea or abdominal pain of 6–12 months. Comorbidities included four cases of ovarian endometriosis, two tubal haematocele, and one adenomyosis. All 11 patients underwent hysteroscopic oblique septum resection, 6 patients had simultaneous laparoscopic surgery, and 6 patients had intraoperative-assisted ultrasound monitoring. Nine patients were followed up for 3–10 years. Among them, one had natural pregnancy, one had a secondary hysterectomy for adenomyosis, and two were intrauterine adhesions and received hysteroscopy. In total, seven patients had normal menstruation without pregnancy.

References

1. Robert H. Asymmetrical bifidities with unilateral menstrual retention (apropos of 12 cases). Chirurgie Memoires Acad Chir. 1970;96(11):769–99.
2. Pfeifer SM, Attaran M, Goldstein J, et al. ASRM Müllerian anomalies classification 2021. Fertil Steril. 2021;116(5):1238–52.
3. Benzineb N, Bellasfar M, Merchaoui J, Sfar R. Robert's uterus with menstrual retention in the blind cavity. J Gynecol Obstet Biol Reprod (Paris). 1993;22(4):366–8.

4. Yang QM, Li H, He SH, Chen D, Chen L. Pregnancy in a blind hemi-cavity of Robert's uterus with ipsilateral renal agenesis: a case report and literature review. J Int Med Res. 2019;47(7):3427–34.
5. Ludwin A, Ludwin I, Bhagavath B, Lindheim SR. Pre-, intra-, and postoperative management of Robert's uterus. Fertil Steril. 2018;110(4):778–9.
6. Takeuchi H, Kitade M, Kikuchi I, Kumakiri J, Kuroda K, Jinushi M. Diagnosis, laparoscopic management, and histopathologic findings of juvenile cystic adenomyoma: a review of nine cases. Fertil Steril. 2010;94(3):862–8.
7. Kiyak H, Karacan T, Wetherilt L, Seckin K, Ozyurek E. Laparoscopic blinded endometrial cavity resection for Robert's uterus. J Minim Invasive Gynecol. 2018;25(2):340.
8. Xia E. Eleven cases Robert's uterus treated by hysteroscopy and laparoscopy successfully delivered in 1 case. J Minim Invasive Gynecol. 2015;22(6s):S192–3.

Chapter 5
Accessory Cavitated Uterine Mass

Zichen Zhao, Shan Deng, and Lan Zhu

Abstract The accessory cavitated uterine mass (ACUM) is a rare obstructive malformation of the female genital tract. It is characterized by a cavitated mass with an inner lining of the endometrium filled with accumulated blood, located under the attachment of the round ligament to the uterus. The patient's uterine cavity, fallopian tubes, and ovaries are normal. Patients with ACUM have clinical manifestations of progressive dysmenorrhea and can be diagnosed with the help of pelvic MRI and transvaginal ultrasonography. Small foci of adenomyosis could be found in the myometrium adjacent to the ACUM, but not in the rest of the uterus. Complete resection of the mass can fully relieve dysmenorrhea.

Keywords Accessory cavitated uterine mass · Round ligament · Dysmenorrhea · Endometrium · Obstructive malformation

The accessory cavitated uterine mass (ACUM) is a rare obstructive malformation of the female genital tract, characterized by a round cavitated mass with an inner lining of the endometrium filled with accumulated blood (Fig. 5.1). It can be found below the attachment of the round ligament to the uterus, sometimes on a lateral side. The pathogenesis of ACUM is still controversial. It is now considered a new type of Müllerian duct anomaly, caused by duplication and persistence of Müllerian duct tissue, possibly related to a gubernaculum dysfunction [1, 2]. The gubernaculum is developed from muscle fibers beyond the Müllerian ducts. Its attachment to the Müllerian ducts induces the fusion of the Müllerian ducts, the full development of the uterus, and the descent of the ovary [3].

Z. Zhao · S. Deng · L. Zhu (✉)
Department of Obstetrics and Gynecology, Peking Union Medical College Hospital, Chinese Academy of Medical Sciences and Peking Union Medical College, Beijing, China

L. Zhu et al. (eds.), *Diagnosis and Management of Female Obstructive Genital Malformations*, https://doi.org/10.1007/978-981-19-6759-7_5

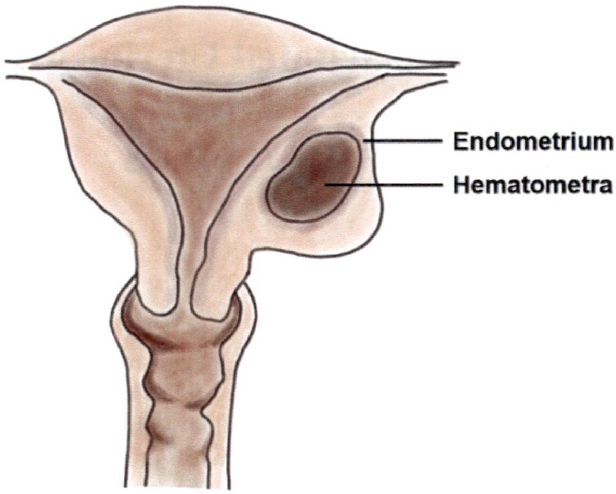

Fig. 5.1 Sectional diagram of ACUM

5.1 Symptoms

Most of the patients with ACUM were nulliparous women, usually younger than 30 years old. They have clinical manifestations of progressive dysmenorrhea, persistent pelvic pain, and abdominal cramps, especially in the unilateral iliac fossa [2]. As ACUM is a congenital malformation, the cyclic exfoliation of the endometrium in the mass cannot be excreted during puberty. Conservative treatment such as NSAIDs or oral contraceptives is not good or effective [1]. But sometimes the patients develop symptoms after childbirth or when they get older [4].

5.2 Physical Examination

A mass in the left or right uterine horn can be palpated by bimanual examination, with tenderness, similar to uterine fibroids [2].

5.3 Complications and Reproductive Outcome

Small foci of adenomyosis could be found in the myometrium adjacent to the accessory cavitated uterine mass but not in the rest of the uterus, probably due to the increased intracavity pressure present during menstruation. It was reported that the risk of uterine rupture would not increase during pregnancy if the uterine cavity was not entered during the resection of the mass [5].

5.4 Diagnosis

5.4.1 Diagnostic Criteria

The diagnostic criteria for ACUM include (1) an isolated accessory cavitated mass located under the round ligament; (2) normal uterus, fallopian tubes, and ovaries (with occasional exceptions [2]); (3) the accessory cavity with an inner lining of the endometrium with glands and stroma, containing chocolate-brown fluid contents; and (4) no adenomyosis or cystic adenomyoma in the rest of the uterus, but small adenomyosis foci can be found in the myometrium adjacent to the ACUM.

The appearance of ACUM under laparoscopy is shown in Fig. 5.2.

5.4.2 Diagnostic Method

The key point of diagnosis is to associate the patient's clinical manifestations with the disease, including the age of onset, the specific location of the mass, and the awareness of its pathological features. When considering the disease, ultrasonography and pelvic MRI are helpful in diagnosis and differential diagnosis [2]. Common diagnostic methods are as follows:

1. Transvaginal (or transrectal) pelvic ultrasonography

   It is the first choice for imaging detection. A mass in the left or right anterior wall of the uterus can be detected, which is similar to the leiomyoma. But unlike uterine fibroids, a cavity can be seen inside the mass, while the endometrium is in situ and the rest of the uterine myometrium are normal.
2. Pelvic MRI

   MRI shows that the ACUM is located in the anterolateral of the uterus or within the broad ligament, and the cavity is not connected to the normal uterine cavity (Fig. 5.3). The high signal intensity in the cavity was observed on

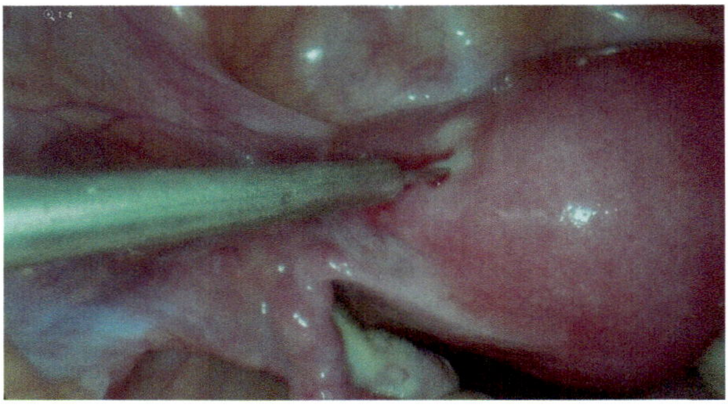

Fig. 5.2 Laparoscopic findings of ACUM

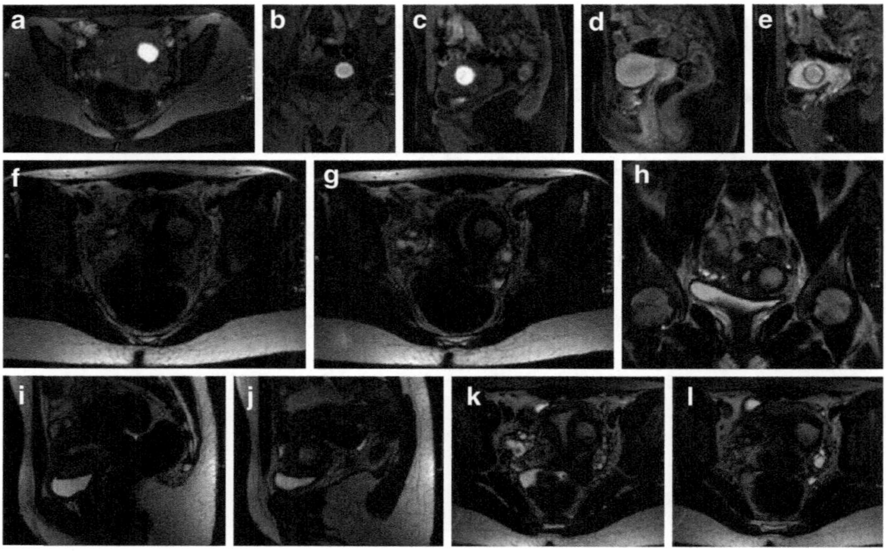

Fig. 5.3 Pelvic MRI in a patient with ACUM. (Copy from Acien et al. [2])

T1-weighted images suggesting hematoma. On T2-weighted images, a low signal surrounding the hematoma was seen, which indicated hemosiderin deposition.

Pelvic MRI shows an accessory endometrial cavity in the left myometrial wall, with hyperintense signals in T1, suggesting hematometra. The lesion is surrounded by a hypointense ring in potentiated sequences of T2, suggesting hemosiderin deposits. (A) T1, transversal cut. (B) T1, coronal cut. (C) T1, sagittal cut. (D and E) T1, sagittal cuts with contrast. (F and G) T2, transversal cuts. (H) T2, coronal cuts. (I) T2, central sagittal cut. (J) T2, left lateral sagittal cut. (K and L) T2, transversal cuts.

3. Hysterosalpingography (HSG)

   The normal uterine cavity and bilateral fallopian tubes can be observed in the patients with ACUM on exploration of HSG, thus distinguishing ACUM from unicornuate uterus complicated with rudimentary horn uterus with functional endometrium (Fig. 5.4). However, the clinical significance of HSG examination is weakening because the shape of the uterus can be detected by MRI already [5].

4. Three-dimensional (3D) ultrasonography

   3D ultrasonography in a coronal section can be used to diagnose ACUM and exclude other malformations of the Müllerian duct. It is more economical and convenient than MRI (Fig. 5.5).

5. Hysteroscopy

   Hysteroscopy clearly shows whether the lesion was submucosal, usually carried out synchronously with laparoscopy (Fig. 5.6).

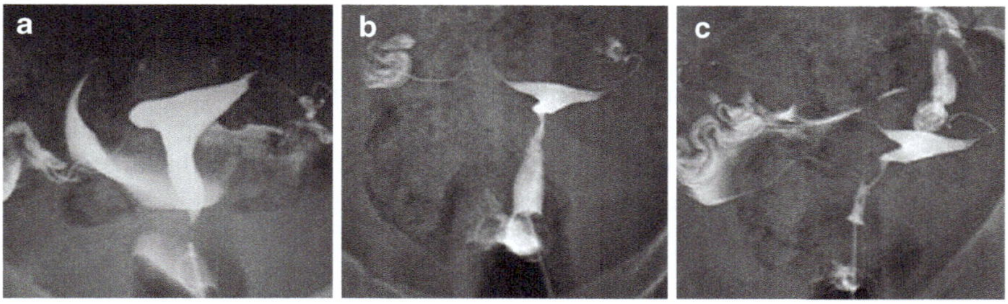

Fig. 5.4 HSG in a patient with ACUM. (Copy from Acién et al. [2])

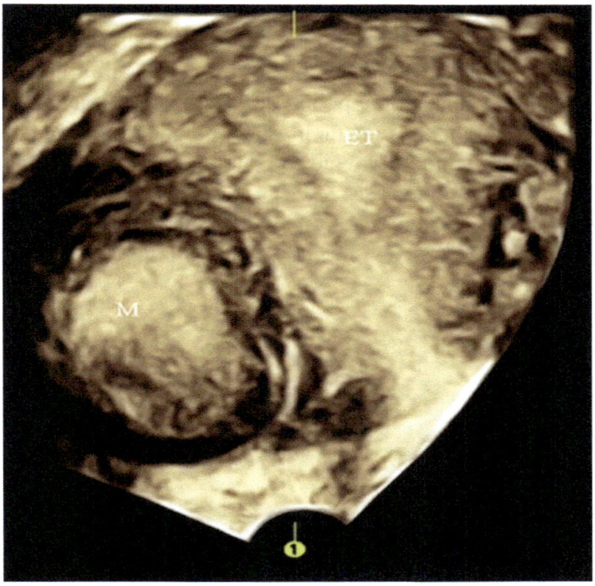

Fig. 5.5 3D ultrasonography in a patient with ACUM3D coronal ultrasound shows a noncommunicating cavitated mass along the right lateral uterine wall below the right cornu. Normal main uterine cavity with both the cornu visualized. (M mass, ET endometrium). (Copy from Shah et al. [6])

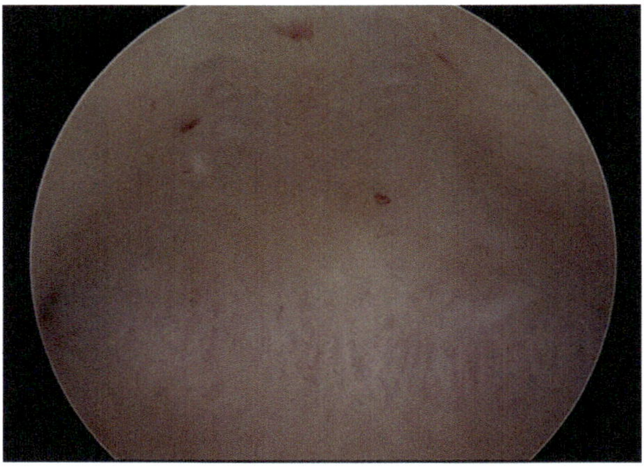

Fig. 5.6 Hysteroscopy in a patient with ACUM: normal uterine cavity and openings of fallopian tubes. (Copy from Paul et al. [3])

5.4.3 Pathological Diagnosis

The gross specimen of the mass is shown in Fig. 5.2, and the histological sections are shown in Fig. 5.7. The covered endometrium on the inner surface of the mass is composed of columnar epithelial cells, glands, and matrix, and the thick peripheral layer is composed of uterine smooth muscle tissue.

5.4.4 Differential Diagnosis

1. Juvenile cystic adenomyoma (JCA)

   At present, the distinction between JCA and ACUM is unclear. Although they are named differently, the clinical and pathological features of the diseases are very similar. Some people think that JCA may be a special type of ACUM [1]. JCA might also occur in other parts of the uterus. More cases are needed for reclassification to avoid overlap of diseases [7].
2. Cystic adenomyosis

   Cystic adenomyosis usually occurs in women of childbearing age with severe adenomyosis backgrounds. The patient's age is usually older than that of the

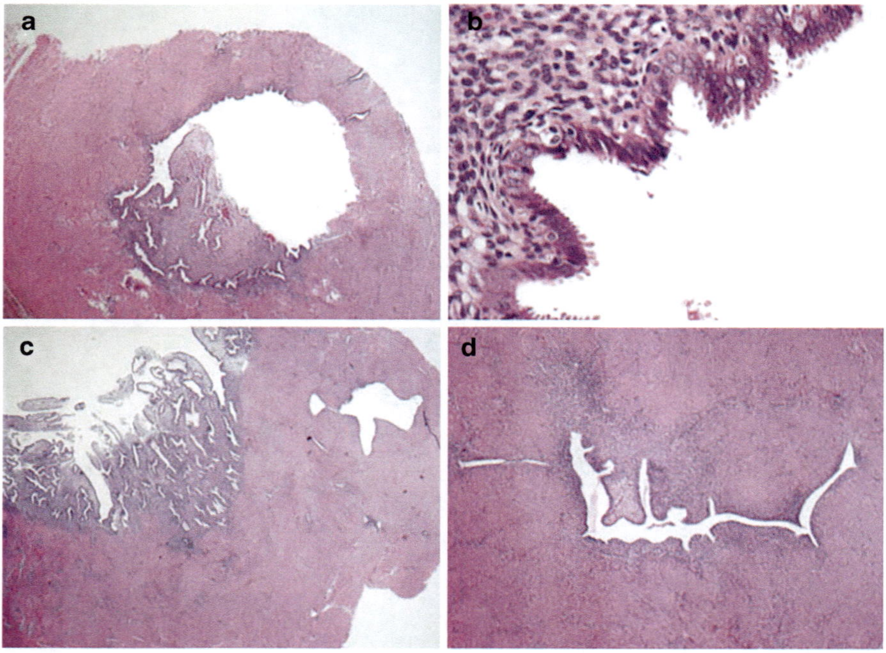

Fig. 5.7 Tissue sections of ACUM specimens stained by hematoxylin and eosin. The magnification from A to D in order is ×4, ×20, ×10, and ×10, respectively. (Copy from Acién et al. [2])

patients with ACUM, and the boundary of the lesion is ambiguous with no special locational characteristics. The endometrial lining and uterine-like structure cannot be found by histopathological examination.

3. Unicornuate uterus complicated with rudimentary horn uterus with functional endometrium

   Normal uterine cavity and uterine horns can be seen in patients with ACUM. However, for patients with unicornuate uterus complicated with rudimentary horn uterus with functional endometrium, the opposite side to the lesion was a unicorn uterus, and the uterine cavity was only connected to the unilateral fallopian tube. Imageology examinations such as MRI and HSG are helpful for preliminary diagnosis, and hysteroscopy combined with laparoscopy is an effective method for differential diagnosis.

4. Uterine leiomyoma with cystic degeneration

   Uterine leiomyoma can have central cystic degeneration but seldom with blood contents. It may occur anywhere in the uterus, not necessarily below the uterine round ligament insertion. And the covered epithelium is not endometrium. The lesion can be single or multiple. Cyclic pain does not usually occur [5].

5.5 Management

The best treatment is complete resection of the mass under laparoscopy or laparotomy. The mass resection is not easy because of the ambiguous boundary of the lesion and the existence of fibrotic tissue near the normal endometrium [2].

All the patients suspected of ACUM who have sexual history should be examined by hysteroscopy to exclude other developmental abnormalities of the Müllerian duct and determine the involvement of submucosal tissue. Then the surgery can be performed under general anesthesia to confirm the diagnosis and resect the lesion.

Because most patients with ACUM are young and need to retain fertility, it is important to close the mass cavity after the resection of the lesion. The boundary of the ACUM is unclear, and the muscle fibers are disordered. Therefore, it is difficult to dissect the partial structure. The operation is recommended to be carried out by doctors with rich experience in laparoscopic resection and suture for complete lesion resection and to reduce the later risk of pregnancy complications.

5.6 Postoperative Management

If there is no complication of endometriosis, no adjuvant medication is needed after the mass resection. If the patient is complicated with endometriosis, medication for endometriosis should be prescribed.

To sum up, ACUM is a rare obstructive developmental anomaly of the Müllerian duct, characterized by severe and early-onset dysmenorrhea at a specific location.

Imaging examination shows cystic intermuscular lesions under the round ligament near the uterine horn, while the uterine cavity and fallopian tubes are normal. Surgical resection is the main treatment. Gaining knowledge of ACUM is helpful to expand the thinking of differential diagnosis and improve the accuracy of diagnosis and treatment.

References

1. Acién P, Acién M, Fernández F, et al. The cavitated accessory uterine mass: a Müllerian anomaly in women with an otherwise normal uterus. Obstet Gynecol. 2010;116(5):1101–9.
2. Acién P, Bataller A, Fernández F, et al. New cases of accessory and cavitated uterine masses (ACUM): a significant cause of severe dysmenorrhea and recurrent pelvic pain in young women. Hum Reprod. 2012;27(3):683–94.
3. Paul PG, Chopade G, Das T, et al. Accessory cavitated uterine mass: a rare cause of severe dysmenorrhea in young women. J Minim Invasive Gynecol. 2015;22(7):1300–3.
4. Putta T, John R, Simon B, et al. Imaging manifestations of accessory cavitated uterine mass – a rare Mullerian anomaly. Indian J Radiol Imaging. 2021;31(3):545–50.
5. Bedaiwy MA, Henry DN, Elguero S, et al. Accessory and cavitated uterine mass with functional endometrium in an adolescent: diagnosis and laparoscopic excision technique. J Pediatr Adolesc Gynecol. 2013;26(4):e89–91.
6. Shah MV, Pisat S, Jain M, et al. Role of 3D coronal ultrasound in diagnosis of accessory and cavitated uterine mass: a rare Mullerian anomaly. J Obstet Gynaecol India. 2021;71(6):633–6.
7. Peyron N, Jacquemier E, Charlot M, et al. Accessory cavitated uterine mass: MRI features and surgical correlations of a rare but under-recognised entity. Eur Radiol. 2019;29(3):1144–52.

Part III
Cervical Malformations

Chapter 6
Congenital Cervical Malformations

Yiying Sun and Lan Zhu

Abstract Congenital cervical malformations (CCMs) are rare obstructive types of female genital tract anomaly caused by bilateral Müllerian fusion abnormalities, and later canalization abnormalities. CCMs are the most challenging cases to manage and were related to poor functional and reproductive prognosis. The evaluation of a patient suspected of CCMs should include a detailed medical history, physical examination, and imaging tests. Pelvic magnetic resonance imaging is recommended for diagnosis and to subclassify the anomaly. Hysterectomy has been the mainstay treatment for CCMs for many decades. With the advancements in surgical techniques and reconstructive materials, conservative surgeries have now been proven to be effective and safe to restore the anatomy, relieve symptoms, and preserve the patients' reproductivity.

Keywords Congenital malformations · Cervical agenesis/dysgenesis · Primary amenorrhea · Conservative surgery

Congenital cervical malformations (CCMs) represent an obstructive anomaly caused by bilateral Müllerian fusion abnormalities and later canalization abnormalities. The prevalence ranges from 1/80,000 to 1/100,000 [1]; in about 50% of cases, they coexist with congenital vaginal agenesis [2].

6.1 Classification

CCMs are previously classified as type IB congenital anomaly according to the American Fertility Society/American Society for Reproductive Medicine (AFS/ASRM) classification [3]. It is currently classified as type C4 malformation

Y. Sun · L. Zhu (✉)
Department of Obstetrics and Gynecology, Peking Union Medical College Hospital, Peking Union Medical College, Chinese Academy of Medical Sciences, Beijing, China

L. Zhu et al. (eds.), *Diagnosis and Management of Female Obstructive Genital Malformations*, https://doi.org/10.1007/978-981-19-6759-7_6

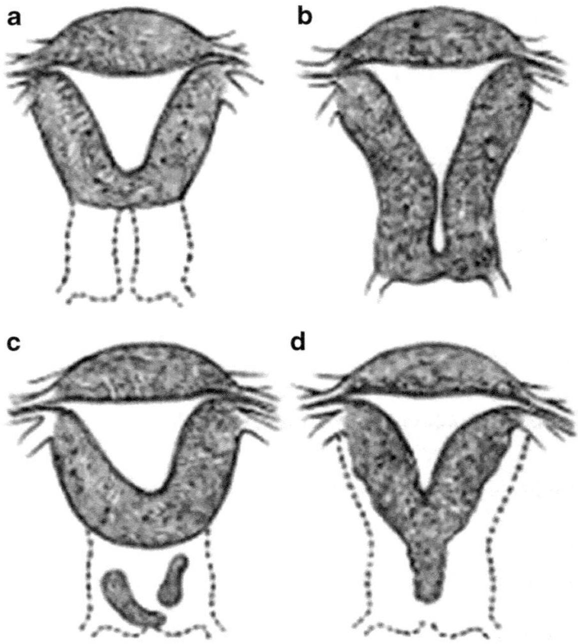

Fig. 6.1 Rocks' classification of cervical malformation. (**a**) Cervical agenesis. (**b**) External cervical os obstruction. (**c**) Cervical fragmentation. (**d**) Cervical fibrous cord. (From [6])

according to the European Society of Human Reproduction and Embryology (ESHRE) and the European Society for Gynecological Endoscopy (ESGE) classification system of female genital tract anomalies [4]. According to Rock's criteria, cervical anomalies can be further classified as cervical aplasia and cervical dysgenesis [5], while the latter can be subclassified as cervical fragmentation, fibrous cord, and cervical obstruction [6] (Fig. 6.1). In cases of cervical fragmentation, separated segments lie within the area of a normal cervix. In cases of cervical fibrous cord, the cervix presents as a fibrous columnar particle with varying diameters. In cases of cervical obstruction, the stroma of the cervix is well-formed, but the external os is obstructed.

6.2 Symptoms

Any pubertal female with primary amenorrhea and symptoms of cyclic abdominal pain should raise the clinical suspicion of congenital cervical malformations. The obstruction of the outflow of menstrual blood may lead to secondary hematometra/hydrometra, hematocolpos/hydrocolpos, and pelvic endometriosis during puberty. The obstructive symptoms may cause psychological burden and loss of productive hours in school and in the life of adolescent girls. Due to the compression of retained blood to adjacent organs, patients may also complain about urinary frequency, dysuria, urinary retention, and difficult defecation. In cases complicated with vaginal atresia, coital intercourse is not possible. In rare cases, patients may be presented with symptoms of acute abdomen [7] and severe pelvic infection.

6.3 Signs

Physical examination is the first step of evaluation. Under the inspection of patients with cervical aplasia, the secondary sex characteristics and appearance of the vulva are normal. In a patient complicated with vaginal atresia, there are no normal vaginal openings, or only a dimple is visible. The well-developed structure of a cervix cannot be palpated, and a cystic mass of retained menstrual blood can be palpated in front of the rectum. If complicated with pelvic inflammatory disease, the cystic mass or lower abdomen may be palpated with tenderness.

6.4 Complications and Reproductive Outcome

Endometriosis and pelvic inflammatory disease secondary to the obstruction of the genital tract are the main complications of congenital cervical malformations. If the obstruction is not relieved over some time, the increasing prevalence of endometriosis is a devastating factor affecting the future normal function of the tubes and the ovaries. Besides, adhesions formed will have a negative impact on surgical approaches.

As congenital cervical malformations indicate poor development and obstruction of the cervical canal and are usually comorbid with vaginal atresia, natural conception is extremely rare for these patients. Secondary endometriosis and pelvic inflammatory disease also hamper patients' fertility. In the past decades, as techniques of conservative surgeries were not mature, most of these patients ended up receiving hysterectomy, and many were deprived of a chance of conception. With the evolution of contemporary surgical techniques and assisted reproductivity technologies, restoration of anatomy and reproductivity preservation have been effectively achieved. According to a systemic review of reproductive outcomes following surgical management of congenital cervical anomalies, 30 pregnancies in 249 patients (12%) were reported, with 27 of those cases being viable pregnancies [8]. Most patients were conceived after in vitro fertilization and transmyometrial embryo transfer and delivered by cesarean section.

6.5 Diagnosis

Based on the clinical history, manifestations, and physical examination, a suspicious diagnosis of obstructive genital tract malformations can be made. Further radiological evaluations are crucial for clarifying the specific anomalies. Pelvic ultrasound (US) may provide reliable, objective, and measurable information about the anatomy of the uterine cervix. The two-dimensional US has a 67.3% sensitivity and a 98.1% specificity, and the three-dimensional US has a 98.3% sensitivity and a 99.4% specificity in diagnosing female genital tract anomalies [4]. However, factors such as the body habitus of the patients and the retroversion of the uterus may compromise obtaining the ideal image.

Magnetic resonance imaging (MRI) has the advantages of high soft-tissue contrast and anatomical resolution, multiplanar imaging capability, and no ionizing radiation. It allows for excellent visualization of reproductive tract anomalies. Compared with a combined laparoscopy and hysteroscopy, MRI can correctly subclassify as many as 85.8% of the cases with female genital tract anomalies [4].

T2-weighted (T2W) images are the most helpful in diagnosing cervical malformations as they can clearly reveal the zonal structures of a well-developed cervix. Four zones can be visualized under MRI. From innermost to outermost, zone 1 is the central hyperintense mucous; zone 2 is the hyperintense endocervical mucosa and glands; zone 3 is the hypointense fibrous stroma; and zone 4 is the loose stroma of intermediate intensity. The absence of four normal zonal structures and an abnormal contour indicates the underdevelopment of a cervix. The four types of cervical malformations have distinct characteristics in MR images (Fig. 6.2). Sagittal T2W images of the long axis of the uterus, cervix, and vagina are the most valuable to show the continuity of genital tract and classify the obstructive genital anomalies. T1-weighted images help show the components of a lesion, such as retained blood, adipose tissue, and so on. In addition, pelvic MRI may also demonstrate complicated extra-genital tract malformations and lesions of endometriosis.

Differential Diagnosis

1. Imperforated hymen: As one of the obstructive anomalies, patients also present with primary amenorrhea and cyclical abdominal pain. The vestibular mucosa appears to be bluish and protrudes outward. A cystic mass can also be palpated in front of the rectum but at a lower location. In radiological tests, the vagina and cervix are normally developed.
2. Vaginal atresia: The symptoms of vaginal atresia are similar to those of cervical anomalies. There is no normal vaginal opening under inspection. Rectal examinations can also palpate a cyst of retained blood above the atretic segment. Radiological imaging shows a complete or partial absence of the vagina, with or without cervical anomalies. The vagina above the atretic part, the cervical canal, and the uterine cavity may be enlarged by retained blood.
3. Secondary atresia of the cervix: Factors like trauma, infection, surgery, and radiotherapy may damage the cervix and cause secondary adhesion of the cervix. Patients who once had regular menstruation can develop symptoms of genital

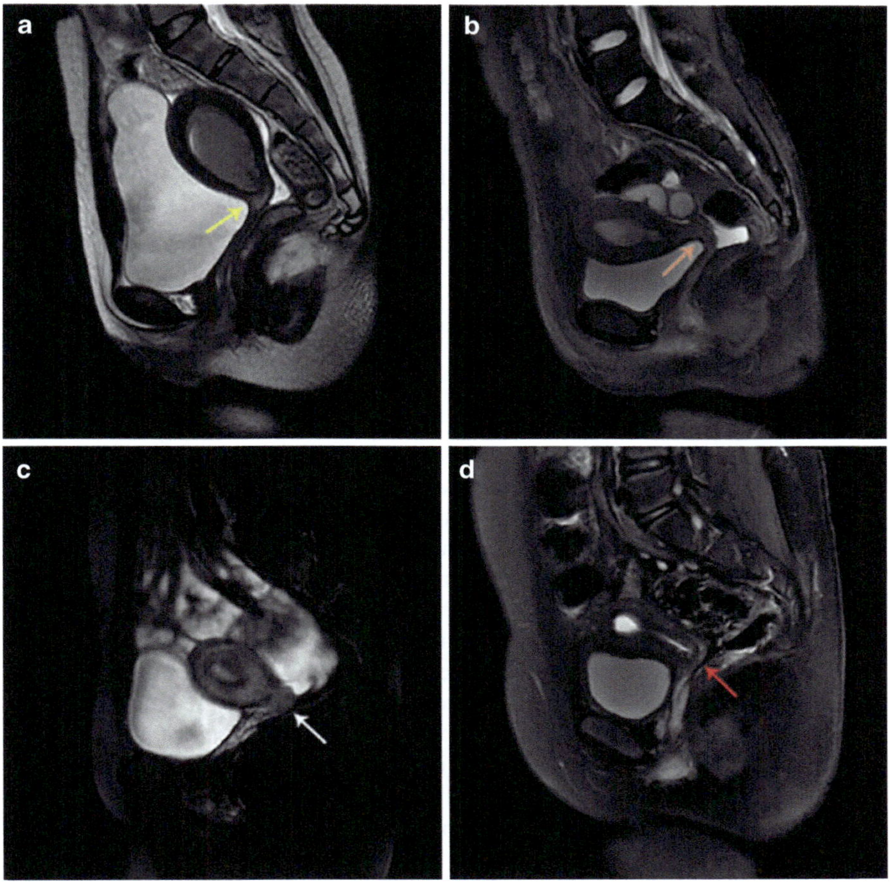

Fig. 6.2 Magnetic resonance imaging findings of various cervical anomalies. (**a**) Cervical agenesis (yellow arrow). (**b**) Cervical fibrous cord (pink arrow). (**c**) Cervical fragmentation (white arrow). (**d**) Cervical obstruction (red arrow)

tract obstruction and inflammation gradually after exogenous injuries to the cervix.

6.6 Management

The management for congenital cervical malformations aims to (1) restore the normal anatomy, (2) relieve the obstructive symptoms, and (3) preserve the uterus for future fertility. As obstruction of the genital tract causes progressive exacerbation of endometriosis and damage to the uterine and ovarian function, management should be implemented once the diagnosis is made and surgery is the primary approach.

6.6.1 Menstrual Suppression

As most cases are initially diagnosed during puberty, an adolescent girl and her family may not be prepared for immediate surgical treatment. As a conservative transient treatment alternative, the continuous use of a contraceptive pill can help control the symptoms and delay the progress of secondary endometriosis. The use of gonadotropin-releasing hormone analogues for a limited time in an adult patient can also provide an alternative treatment so long as the appropriate add-back therapy is offered to the patient.

6.6.2 Surgical Treatment

The initial experiences of conservative surgeries for treating congenital cervical malformations are not satisfactory. Conservative surgeries may lead to injuries to adjacent organs. Even after restoring the anatomy, the patients may still experience refractory restenosis of the genital tract and secondary pelvic inflammatory disease. Thus, hysterectomy has been the mainstay of treatments for congenital cervical malformations for many decades. Even today, for cases complicated with severe endometriosis, pelvic adhesions, or infections and those with severe uterine malformation, hysterectomy may still be considered a rational choice. However, the iatrogenic menopause and loss of reproductive function can cause great damage to the social and psychological function of the patients after the extirpative surgery. With the great advancements in surgical techniques and biological materials, conservative surgeries have now proven to be effective and safe to restore the anatomy, relieve symptoms, and preserve the patients' reproductivity [5].

6.6.2.1 Preoperative Preparation

1. Comprehensive assessment: Before determining the type of surgery, physicians should consider factors that influence the risks and benefits of surgery: the type of cervical malformations, the presence or absence of a vagina, the complicated genital tract anomalies, and the severity of endometriosis. Collaboration with radiological physicians in reviewing the pelvic ultrasound and MRI images may help delineate the anatomic features.
2. Preoperative counseling and explanation of the surgery: The possible intraoperative and postoperative risks and complications should be thoroughly discussed with the patients and their guardians (if applicable), issues including the possible surgical risk of injuries to adjacent organs, risk of failure of conservative surgery, need of long-term follow-up after surgery, the possibility of future restenosis, infection, and hysterectomy in the short or long future. The pros and cons of conservative and extirpative surgical options should be discussed.

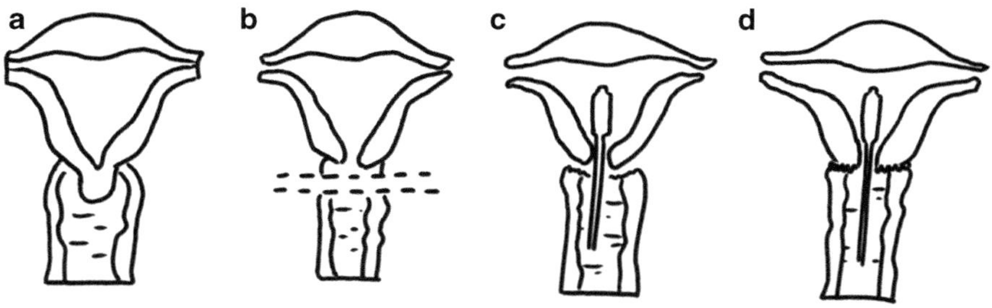

Fig. 6.3 Schematic illustration of uterovaginal anastomosis. (**a**) Congenital cervical atresia before surgical correction. (**b**) Resection of the atretic cervix. (**c**) A Foley catheter is inserted transvaginally into the endometrial cavity and anchored. (**d**) The lower segment of the uterus is anastomosed to the upper vaginal mucosa with interrupted sutures

3. Preoperative preparation: Prophylactic antibiotics are recommended, especially for patients complicated by pelvic inflammatory disease. Bowel preparation may help expose a wider surgical field and minimize incisional contamination.

6.6.2.2 Key Technical Points

Direct Uterovaginal Anastomosis or Cervical Vaginal Anastomosis
This technique is suitable for cases of cervical agenesis or cases with little remnants of the cervix that are hard to canalize. It requires adequate dissection of the utero-vesical and rectouterine pouch, resection of the poorly developed cervix, pulling down the lower segment of the uterus, and anastomosis to the vaginal or vestibule mucosa. The schematic illustration is shown in Fig. 6.3. With laparoscopy or laparotomy, a probe is inserted into the uterine cavity to identify the lowermost portion of the uterine cavity. Another probe is then inserted trans-vaginally to identify the topmost portion of the atretic part. The atretic tissue of the cervix can then be resected abdominally. A Foley catheter is inserted trans-vaginally into the uterine cavity and anchored with a water balloon. The lower segment of the uterus is interruptedly sutured to the vaginal or vestibule mucosa with absorbable stitches. The intrauterine catheter is kept in situ to prevent restenosis soon after the surgery.

Direct Uterovaginal Canalization or Cervicovaginal Canalization
If sufficient cervical stroma is present, canalization can attempt to create a channel through the atretic cervix. In contrast to the above direct uterovaginal anastomosis approach, there is no need to dissect the vesico/recto-uterine pouch, so this technique is comparatively easy to conduct, and the risk of postoperative pelvic adhesion is lower. However, for cases with narrow vesico-uterine space and a solid cervical remnant, it is difficult to canalize successfully, and there is a risk of damaging the adjacent organs. The procedure includes (Fig. 6.4) [9] the following: step 1: laparoscopic inspection of the uterus, bilateral adnexa, and pelvis; step 2: an incision is made at the anterior wall of the uterus. A metal guide is then pushed

downward from the incision to guide the lowest portion of the uterus; step 3: a metal catheter in front and a finger behind can guide the direction of the urethra and rectum, respectively. Another finger bluntly dissects the space between the urethra and rectum to create a channel. With a finger directing the lowermost part of the atretic cervix in the vagina, the metal guide in the uterine cavity is pushed downward and canalizes the atretic cervical stroma; step 4: a Foley catheter is dragged from the vagina upward and anchored in the uterine cavity; step 5: the incision at the anterior wall of the uterus was closed by absorbable stitches; and step 6: the catheter was sutured to the canalized cervix for fixation.

Reconstructive surgeries aim to restore the continuity of the vagina, cervix, and uterus, but preserving the postoperative patency remains a challenging issue in this territory. To prevent adhesion and promote epithelialization of the reconstructed cervix, various grafts and materials have been clinically used, e.g., small intestinal submucosa (SIS) graft, split or full-thickness skin graft, peritoneal flap, vaginal mucosa, polytetrafluoroethylene (PTFE) graft, etc. A common approach is to wrap the epithelial material into a cylinder shape over a stent or a Foley tube, which is inserted and fixed to the newly formed canal to cover the rough area. However, there is still no consensus on which material is better. A systemic review indicated that the full-thickness skin graft was statistically associated with poor outcomes in terms of

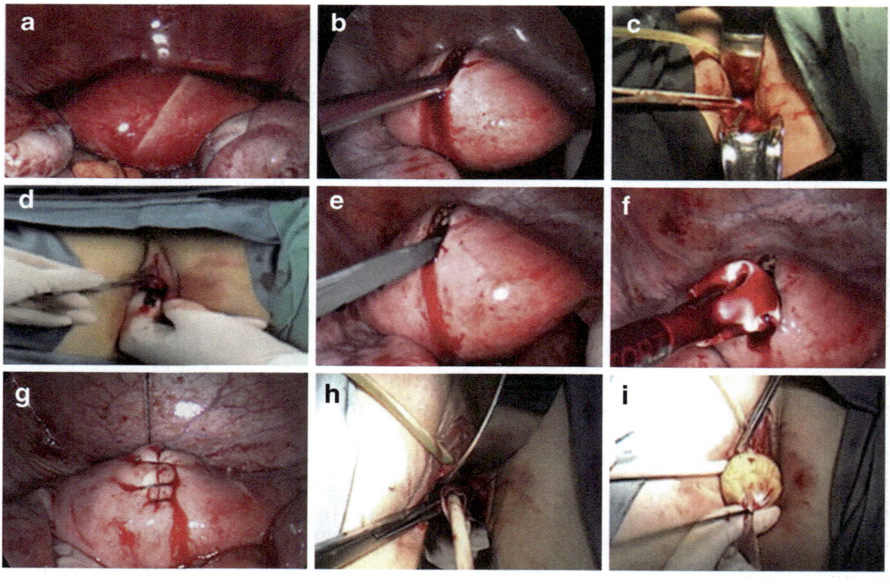

Fig. 6.4 Surgical procedures of uterovaginal canalization. (**a**) Inspection of pelvic cavity. (**b**) An incision is made at the anterior wall of the uterus and a metal guide is pushed downward. (**c**) A channel was created with blunt dissection between the urethra and the rectum. (**d**) The lowermost of the atretic segment is canalized. (**e**, **f**) A mushroom-like catheter is dragged upward to the uterine cavity. (**g**) The uterine incision is closed. (**h**) The catheter is anchored to the cervix. (**i**) A soft mold is placed in the vagina

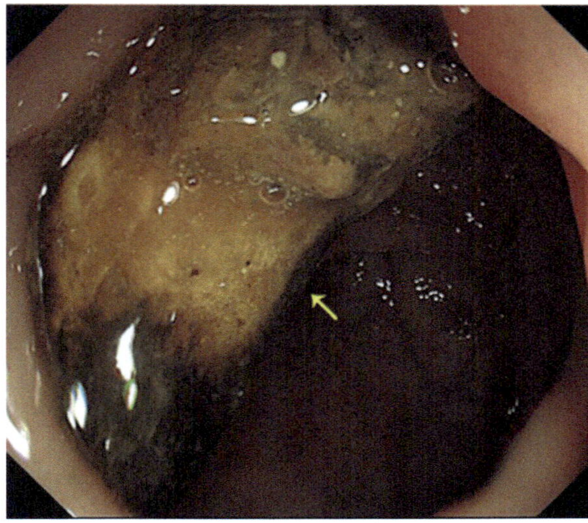

Fig. 6.5 Migration of drainage tube to the rectum after reconstructive surgery

menstruation restoration and the need for hysterectomy after this reconstructive surgery [8].

To prevent collapse and stenosis of the created canal, most physicians choose to place drainage tubes or stents in situ. Foley tubes and their derivatives are the most applied devices considering their good compatibility and patency advantages. Besides, silicon and nickel-titanium stents are also used. The durability of the tubes is not consistent as reported in the literature, varying from a few weeks to years. However, the patency and location of the stent should be regularly evaluated and removed at the proper time. A case was reported that a girl was presented to the emergency room, 4 years after this reconstructive surgery, with vaginal defecation and periodic severe lower abdominal pain. Colonoscopy and laparotomy revealed that the Pezzer catheter migrated and caused a rectovaginal fistula (Fig. 6.5) [10].

6.6.2.3 Postoperative Management and Follow-Up

1. Intravenous antibiotics are recommended to prevent genital tract infections. Patients who are complicated by pelvic infection or have received an emergent surgery may be prescribed an upgraded regimen.
2. For patients who received a vaginoplasty, a soft mold made of gauze is usually placed to prevent bleeding and adhesion. A Foley catheter can be maintained for a few days until the mold is taken out. Laxative can be prescribed to avoid traction to the surgical wound during difficult bowel movement.
3. Postoperative fluid and nutrition supply should be consulted with pediatrics as most patients are in their teens.

4. A vaginal mold is used and changed regularly until complete healing of the vaginal epithelium. If there is no expected sex life, the mold should be used regularly for 6–24 months to reduce the incidence of postoperative vaginal stenosis.
5. Follow-up: Conservative surgery is just the start of the reconstructive management. The possible complications of restenosis and retrograde infections necessitate comprehensive patient education and regular follow-up. The first visit could be arranged in the third month after the operation to evaluate wound healing and patients' self-care. The following visits, with 6–12 months intervals, involve testing of serum CA 125 level, pelvic ultrasound, and checking of patency of tubes or stents.

References

1. Fujimoto VY, Miller JH, Klein NA, Soules MR. Congenital cervical atresia: report of seven cases and review of the literature. Am J Obstet Gynecol. 1997;177(6):1419.
2. Grimbizis GF. Successful end-to-end cervico-cervical anastomosis in a patient with congenital cervical fragmentation: case report. Hum Reprod. 2004;19(5):1204–10.
3. The American Fertility Society classifications of adnexal adhesions, distal tubal occlusion, tubal occlusion secondary to tubal ligation, tubal pregnancies, Müllerian anomalies and intrauterine adhesions. Fertil Steril. 1988;49(6):944–55.
4. Grimbizis GF, Gordts S, Di Spiezio Sardo A, et al. The ESHRE/ESGE consensus on the classification of female genital tract congenital anomalies. Hum Reprod. 2013;28(8):2032–44.
5. Mikos T, Gordts S, Grimbizis GF. Current knowledge about the management of congenital cervical malformations: a literature review. Fertil Steril. 2020;113(4):723–32.
6. Rock JA, Roberts CP, Jones HW. Congenital anomalies of the uterine cervix: lessons from 30 cases managed clinically by a common protocol. Fertil Steril. 2010;94(5):1858–63.
7. Omurtag K, Session D, Brahma P, Matlack A, Roberts C. Horizontal uterine torsion in the setting of complete cervical and partial vaginal agenesis: a case report. Fertil Steril. 2009;91(5):1957.e13–5.
8. Mikos T, Lantzanaki M, Anthoulakis C, Grimbizis GF. Functional and reproductive outcomes following surgical management of congenital anomalies of the cervix: a systematic review. J Minim Invasive Gynecol. 2021;28(8):1452–61.e16.
9. Kang J, Chen N, Zhang Y, et al. Laparoscopically assisted uterovaginal canalization and vaginoplasty for patients with congenital cervical and vaginal atresia: a step-by-step guide and long-term outcomes. J Minim Invasive Gynecol. 2021;28(6):1203–10.
10. Kang J, Zhu L. Migration of cervical stent after cervico-vaginal canalization. Int Urogynecol J. 2020;31(6):1281.

Part IV
Obstructive Vaginal Malformations

Chapter 7
Vagina Atresia

Yiying Sun and Lan Zhu

Abstract Vagina atresia is a rare congenital genital tract anomaly caused by abnormal development of the urogenital sinus and the caudal part of the Müllerian ducts during embryonic development. It is characterized by partial or complete absence of the vagina, with usually well-developed and functional uterus. The incidence of congenital absence of vagina is 1/4000 to 1/5000, of which only 7–8% were vaginal atresia associated with normal uterus. Vaginal atresia is one of the obstructive genital tract malformations causing typical symptoms of primary amenorrhea, cyclical lower abdominal pain, and pelvic mass. Conservative surgical corrections are fundamental approaches relieving the symptoms and preserving the patients' fertility reservation.

Keywords Vaginal atresia · Obstructive genital tract malformations · Vaginoplasty

7.1 Classification

The embryologic origin of the vagina is controversial, but the widely accepted theory is the dual origin theory: the upper 1/3 of the vagina develops from the primordial vagina and the lower 2/3 from the sinovaginal bulb. Vaginal atresia is defined as the V4 malformations according to the ESHRE/ESGE classification [1]. Peking Union Medical College Hospital (PUMCH) further subclassified vaginal atresia into the following two types, based on the portion of the atresia and the concomitant cervical malformation [2] (Fig. 7.1).

Type I vaginal atresia (distal vaginal atresia): The distal portion of the vagina is atretic, while the proximal portion of the vagina, the cervix, and uterine body are well developed.

Y. Sun · L. Zhu (✉)
Department of Obstetrics and Gynecology, Peking Union Medical College Hospital, Peking Union Medical College, Chinese Academy of Medical Sciences, Beijing, China

L. Zhu et al. (eds.), *Diagnosis and Management of Female Obstructive Genital Malformations*, https://doi.org/10.1007/978-981-19-6759-7_7

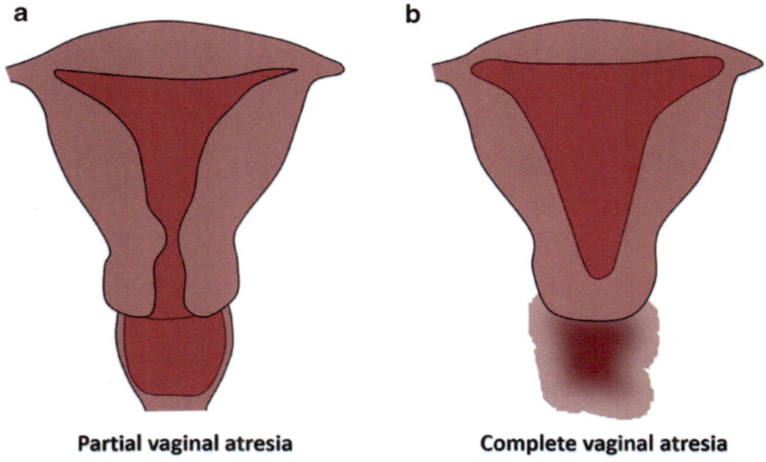

Fig. 7.1 The classification of vaginal atresia. (**a**) Type I vaginal atresia. (**b**) Type II vaginal atresia

Type II vaginal atresia (i.e., complete vaginal atresia): The vagina is completely atretic, usually complicated with cervical aplasia or agenesis.

7.2 Symptoms

Vaginal atresia is an obstructive genital tract abnormality. Due to the obstruction of the genital tract and accumulation of menstrual blood above the atretic segment, these patients present with primary amenorrhea, periodic lower abdominal pain, and pelvic masses. The compression of accumulated menstrual blood on adjacent organs may cause urinary frequency, dysuria, urinary retention, and difficult defecation. Additionally, if the obstruction is not relieved in time, secondary pelvic endometriosis may lead to chronic pelvic pain.

7.3 Signs

Type I vaginal atresia: The vulva is normal in appearance, but there is no vaginal opening in the vestibule. In contrast to imperforate hymen, the lowest portion of the atretic segment is pink and does not bulge outward. During the "menstruation period," the high-tension mass can be palpated anterior to the rectum, and the bottom of the mass is lower compared to that of type II vaginal atresia, but does not reach the level of the hymen (Fig. 7.2).

Type II vaginal atresia: The vulvar presentation is the same as that of type I vaginal atresia (Fig. 7.2). Type II vaginal atresia is often complicated with cervical

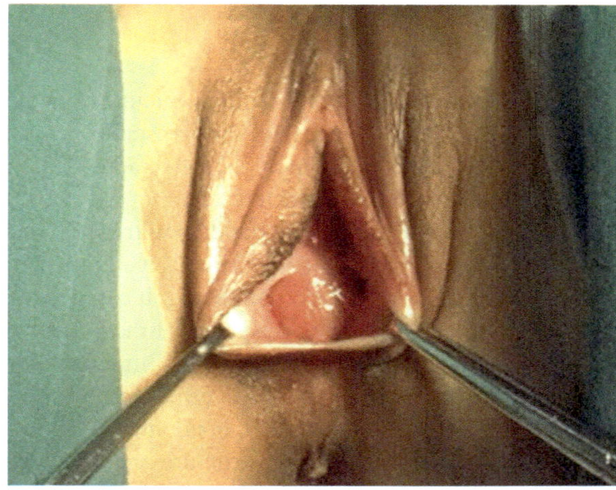

Fig. 7.2 The inspection of the perineum of patients with vaginal atresia

aplasia and in some cases with an underdeveloped uterine body. The cervical canal and uterine cavity are usually enlarged due to the accumulation of blood in the uterine cavity, so a high-tension mass can be palpated anterior to the rectum, and the underdeveloped cervix can also be touched by rectal examination.

7.4 Complications and Pregnancy Outcome

The natural conception is rare for patients with vaginal atresia. The obstruction of the genital tract and secondary pelvic endometriosis may progressively hamper patients' fertility reservation. With the advancement of reconstructive surgical techniques, pregnancy has become realistic for patients with vaginal atresia, mostly achieved by assisted reproductive technology, and term pregnancies have been reported [3, 4]. The pregnancy outcomes are poorer for type II vaginal atresia; the complicated cervical atresia is associated with an increasing risk of restenosis, cervical insufficiency, spontaneous abortion, and preterm birth.

7.5 Diagnosis

Pelvic ultrasound and MRI are useful for preoperative diagnosis and evaluation. If necessary, laparoscopic exploration can help clarify the concomitant cervical and uterine abnormalities as well as pelvic endometriosis.

7.5.1 Diagnostic Methods

1. Pelvic ultrasound: This is the initial diagnostic method as it is easy to perform, inexpensive, and noninvasive. The absence of partial or complete vagina is observed, and hematocolpos, hematotrachelos, and hematometra above the atretic segment may be detected.
2. Urological ultrasound: Since patients with Müllerian anomalies are more likely to have a combination of abnormal development of the urinary tract, routine urological ultrasound is recommended. It can detect abnormalities of the urinary system, such as absence or dysplasia of the kidney and ectopic kidney.
3. Pelvic MRI: With the advantage of the high soft-tissue contrast and multiplanar imaging capability, pelvic MRI is effective and safe to delineate the structure of the vagina, cervix, and detect concomitant anomalies. Sagittal T2-weighted images of the long axis of the structure are most valuable to show the continuity of the genital tract and differentiate the obstructive genital anomalies. The pelvic MRI imaging of vaginal atresia is shown in Fig. 7.3.
4. X-rays and CT: They are valuable for the exclusion of coexisting skeletal system malformations. Complex urinary system anomalies can also be clarified with retrograde pyelography.

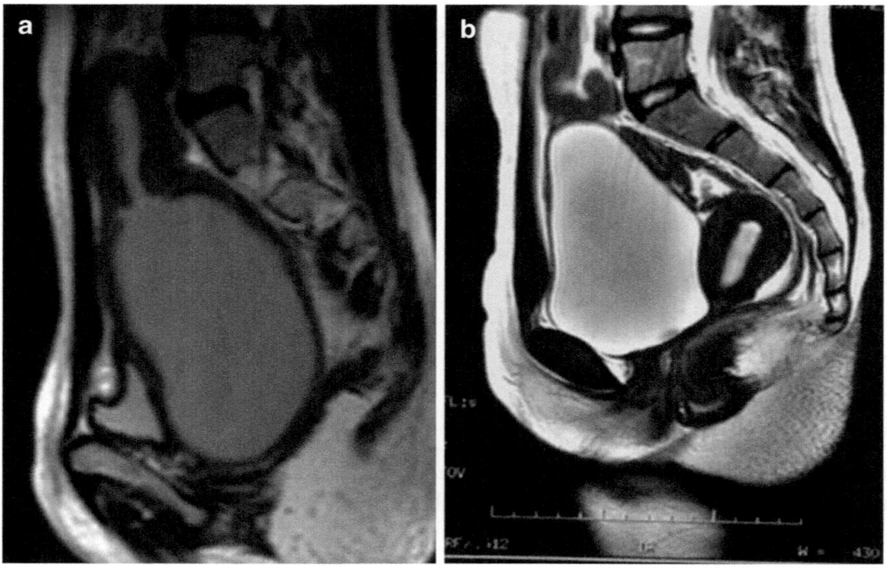

Fig. 7.3 MRI imaging of type I and type II vaginal atresia. (**a**) Type I vaginal atresia. (**b**) Type II vaginal atresia

7.5.2 *Differential Diagnosis*

1. Mayer-Rokintansky-Kuster-Hauser (MRKH) syndrome: MRKH syndrome is caused by bilateral Müllerian duct hypoplasia. Similar to vaginal atresia, MRKH is found with congenital absence of the vagina, while the uterus is absent or present as a primordial uterus. Primary amenorrhea is also the typical symptom of MRKH syndrome, but in contrast to vaginal atresia, most of the cases are free of periodic abdominal pain and pelvic mass, considering the uterus is absent or nonfunctional. Under physical examination, there is no normal vaginal opening in the vestibular area or it is only observed as a shallow dimple, whereas a high-tension mass will not be palpated by rectal examination as there is always no retained menstrual blood. Additionally, the uterus is not present in contrast to a well-developed, sometimes up-floating or enlarged uterus in patients with vaginal atresia. Pelvic ultrasound and magnetic resonance imaging can help differentiate the diagnosis.
2. Imperforate hymen: The hymen is the embryologic septum between the urogenital sinus and sinovaginal bulb and is the distal boundary of the vaginal plate. Patients are similarly presented with primary amenorrhea and cyclical abdominal pain. The typical sign of imperforate hymen is the bluish bulge protruding from the level of hymen, while the lower border of the bulge is lower than that of vaginal atresia. If the bulge is not visible when patients are doing Valsalva, transverse vaginal septum or distal vaginal agenesis should be suspected. Physical examination, pelvic ultrasound, and MRI can assist in the diagnosis.
3. Transverse vaginal septum: It is caused by incomplete canalization at the junction of the Müllerian duct and the urogenital sinus during embryonic development. The septum can be located anywhere in the vagina, but the upper-and-middle junction is the most common. The lower, unperforated vaginal septum has similar symptoms and signs to distal vaginal atresia, which can be distinguished by physical examination, radiologic tests, and surgical exploration.

7.6 Treatment

Surgery is the fundamental approach to relieve genital tract obstruction, prevent progressing pelvic endometriosis, and preserve the patients' reproductive function. For patients with obstructive symptoms after puberty, early surgical treatment is recommended after definitive diagnosis, with the principles of relieving obstruction, reconstructing the vagina, and preventing readhesion.

7.6.1 Type I Vaginal Atresia

The distal segment of the vagina is absent in patients with type I vaginal atresia, while the proximal vaginal tissue is normal. Therefore, vaginoplasty is comparatively easier and safer in patients with partial vaginal atresia. Reconstructive surgery is not required to be performed during menstruation, while for those with hematocolpos, the operation should be performed as soon as possible to relieve the obstruction (Fig. 7.4).

(a) Puncture: Menstruation is an ideal time for surgery as the retained blood above the atretic segment dilates the narrow space between the urethra and rectum. A metal catheter inserted in the urethra and a finger placed in the rectum are helpful to direct the position of the adjacent organs and prevent injuries. A 16G needle can be used to puncture the atretic segment until the retained blood is drained and aspirated, indicating the correct direction of canalization.
(b) Incision: Under the direction of the puncture needle, the atretic lower vaginal segment is incised with a cold or electric knife until more retained blood flows out and the normal upper vaginal cavity is visible.
(c) Dilation and drainage: The canal of puncture is then dilated by the operator's fingers until it can accommodate two fingers. This process is also guided by the metal urethral metal catheter and fingers placed in the rectum to avoid damage

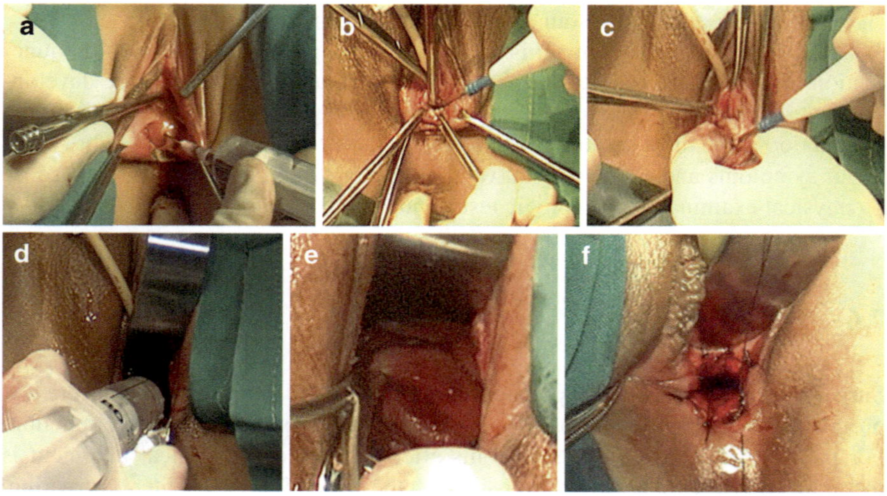

Fig. 7.4 Surgical procedures of vaginoplasty correcting type I vaginal atresia. (**a**) A 16G needle can be used to puncture the atretic segment until the retained blood is drained. (**b**) Incision is made at the lowermost part of the atretic tissue. (**c**) The atretic tissue is removed, and the canal of puncture is then dilated by the operator's fingers until it can accommodate two fingers. (**d**) The created canal is irrigated with saline. (**e**) Inspect the development of the cervix. (**f**) The vestibular mucosa should be pulled up and intermittently sutured with absorbable stitches for fixation to cover the newly created lower vagina

to the adjacent organs. After the vagina is created, the cervix can be clearly visualized, and its development should be inspected clearly to decide on the subsequent method to restore the continuity of vagina and cervix. The upper segment of the vagina should be irrigated with saline or iodine, and the retained blood needs to be adequately drained off.

(d) Prevention of adhesions and promotion of epithelialization: The atretic tissue should be completely removed by electric or cold knife. The vestibular mucosa should be pulled up and intermittently sutured with absorbable stitches for fixation to cover the new-created lower vagina. Skin flap, small intestinal submucosa (SIS) graft, polytetrafluoroethylene (PTFE) graft, etc. have been reported as reconstructed materials preventing postoperative restenosis.

(e) After the completion of vaginoplasty, a soft mold (made by sterile condom or gauze) is placed in situ to stop bleeding by compression. The soft mold is removed and replaced with a rigid mold a few days later. The wound of the created vaginal segment should be examined for healing, and the patient is instructed to place the solid mold regularly to prevent adhesions.

7.6.2 Type II Vaginal Atresia

The surgical correction of type II vaginal atresia is comparatively more difficult considering the complete absence of vagina, the narrow cysto-rectal space, and the complicated cervical anomalies. Therefore, type II vaginal atresia is extremely difficult to manage clinically, and the choice of treatment needs to be decided according to individualized situation. Hysterectomy may be considered in cases complicated with complex uterine and cervical malformations, severe endometriosis, and pelvic infection, or the patients who refuse to take the risk of postoperative complications. The reconstructive surgery is recommended to be performed during menstruation, when menstrual blood dilates the uterine cavity, cervical canal, and atretic tissues.

The key to vaginoplasty is to determine the direction of the atretic vaginal segment and to create a cavity in the vesico-rectal space while avoiding damage to the surrounding organs. The steps of vaginoplasty are similar to the procedure of type I vaginal atresia (Fig. 7.5), which requires careful separation of the connective tissue in the vesicorectal space. Under the direction of a metal catheter inserted in the urethra and a finger guided in the rectum, the space should be bluntly separated to a width of two fingers. In cases of concomitant cervical dysplasia, the method to reconstruct the uterine, cervical, and vaginal continuity should be performed according to the exact type of cervical development (refer to the chapter on cervical dysplasia for details).

To avoid postoperative adhesions of the reconstructed vagina, a variety of materials are used to cover the wound and promote epithelialization. Currently, the most common vaginoplasty procedure used by gynecologists in the United States is the Abbe-McIndoe method [5]. After separation of the vesicorectal space, a mold

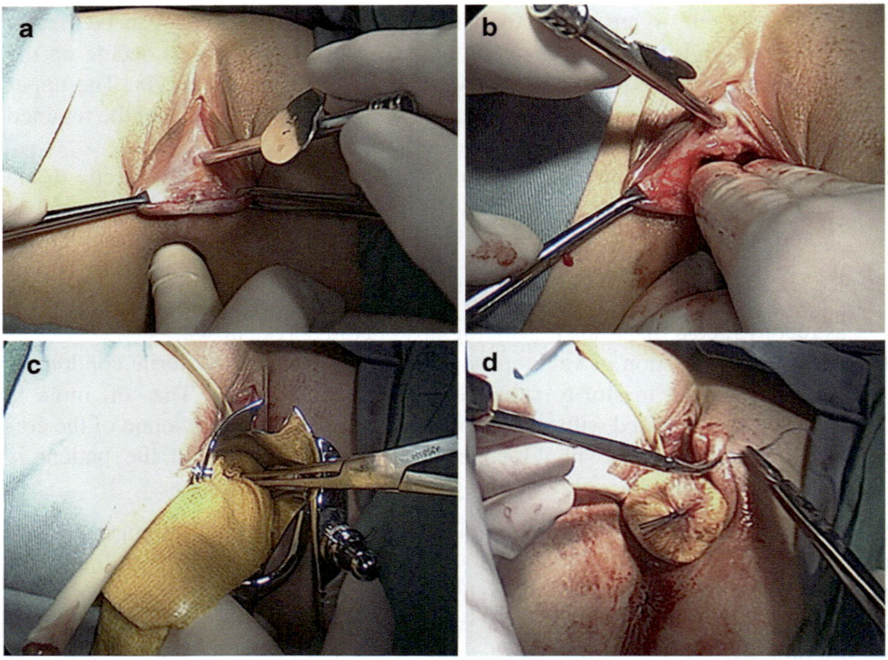

Fig. 7.5 Key point of vaginoplasty correcting type II vaginal atresia. (**a**) A metal catheter inserted in the urethra and a finger placed in the rectum are helpful to direct the position of the adjacent organs and prevent injuries. (**b**) The new vagina is created out of the atretic soft tissue by blunt dissection by fingers. (**c**) The canal can be covered by biomaterials to promote epithelialization and prevent adhesion. (**d**) A soft mold is placed to prevent adhesion and then changed for silicone mold

covered with a split-thickness skin graft is inserted into the formed vagina, and the patient is instructed to insist on self-dilation of the vagina after the procedure. Due to the long-term sebaceous secretion and high restenosis rate after McIndoe's method [6], several modified procedures have been proposed for vaginal reconstruction, such as the use of peritoneal (Davydov), amniotic, peritoneal, polylactic acid prothesis [7], porcine small intestine submucosal biopatch [8], and Interceed. However, there is still no consensus on which is the superior procedure [9].

After the vaginoplasty procedure, the urethral catheter is retained for 1 week to avoid postoperative urinary retention, and intravenous antibiotics are used to prevent postoperative infections. The soft vaginal mold can be replaced by a rigid mold (plastic, silicone texture) 1 week after the operation. Vaginal molds should be placed frequently for at least 3–6 months until the created vagina is completely epithelialized, after which the patients may intermittently self-dilate the vagina until regular sex is achieved.

In conclusion, vaginal atresia is a rare congenital malformation of the female genitourinary system that is characterized by symptoms related to obstruction of the menstrual flow and is prone to secondary infections and endometriosis. Surgical correction of the obstruction is the most fundamental treatment, and clinical management of type II vaginal atresia is difficult and requires individualized decisions.

References

1. Grimbizis GF, Gordts S, Di Spiezio Sardo A, et al. The ESHRE/ESGE consensus on the classification of female genital tract congenital anomalies. Hum Reprod. 2013;28(8):2032–44. https://doi.org/10.1093/humrep/det098.
2. Leng J, Lang J, Lian L, Huang R, Liu Z, Sun D, et al. Congenital vaginal atresia: report of 16 cases. Zhonghua Fu Chan Ke Za Zhi. 2002;37:217–9.
3. Acien P, Acien MI, Quereda F, Santoyo T. Cervicovaginal agenesis: spontaneous gestation at term after previous reimplantation of the uterine corpus in a neovagina: case report. Hum Reprod. 2008;23(3):548–53. https://doi.org/10.1093/humrep/dem420.
4. Chakravarty B, Konar H, Chowdhury NNR. Pregnancies after reconstructive surgery for congenital cervicovaginal atresia. Am J Obstet Gynecol. 2000;183(2):421–3. https://doi.org/10.1067/mob.2000.105740.
5. ACOG Committee on Adolescent Health Care. ACOG Committee Opinion. Number 274, July 2002. Nonsurgical diagnosis and management of vaginal agenesis. Obstet Gynecol. 2002;100(1) https://doi.org/10.1016/s0029-7844(02)02158-0.
6. Rock JA, Roberts CP, Jones HW. Congenital anomalies of the uterine cervix: lessons from 30 cases managed clinically by a common protocol. Fertil Steril. 2010;94(5):1858–63. https://doi.org/10.1016/j.fertnstert.2009.10.024.
7. Navarro V, Acién MI, Acién P. Classical McIndoe technique versus the McIndoe technique with a neovaginal PACIENA Prosthesis® and no skin graft. JCM. 2020;9(11):3648. https://doi.org/10.3390/jcm9113648.
8. Ding Y, Zhang X, Zhang Y, Shen F, Ding J, Hua K. Cervicovaginal reconstruction with small intestinal submucosa graft in congenital cervicovaginal atresia: a report of 38 cases. Eur J Obstet Gynecol Reprod Biol. 2021;267:49–55. https://doi.org/10.1016/j.ejogrb.2021.10.015.
9. Callahan TL, Caughey AB. Blueprints obstetrics & gynecology. Philadelphia: Wolters Kluwer Health/Lippincott William & Wilkins; 2009.

Chapter 8
Herlyn-Werner-Wunderlich Syndrome

Shuang Song, Na Chen, and Lan Zhu

Abstract Herlyn-Werner Wunderlich Syndrome (HWWS) is a rare urogenital tract malformation disease, characterized by uterine didelphys, obstructed hemivagina, and ipsilateral renal anomalies. It is also been named obstructed hemivagina and ipsilateral renal anomaly (OHVIRA) syndrome or oblique vaginal septum syndrome (OVSS). This disease can be classified into four subtypes according to its anatomical features and the extent of menstrual obstruction. Patients will display various symptoms such as pelvic pain, abnormal vaginal discharge, or compression symptoms. The diagnosis of HWWS can be made by pelvic examination and proper imaging methods including ultrasound and MRI. Vaginal septum resection surgery is the most effective treatment method to relieve obstruction, prevent complications, and preserve fertility.

Keywords Herlyn-Werner-Wunderlich syndrome · HWWS · OHVIRA · Oblique vaginal septum syndrome · OVSS · Classification · Treatment

Herlyn-Werner-Wunderlich Syndrome (HWWS) is a rare congenital malformation of the female genitourinary system, characterized by uterine didelphys, obstructed hemivagina, and ipsilateral renal anomalies. Though ipsilateral renal agenesis is the most common renal anomaly, other malformations such as ectopic kidney, polycystic kidney, and repeating collecting system have also been reported in the literature [1, 2]. This syndrome has also been named obstructed hemivagina and ipsilateral renal anomaly (OHVIRA) syndrome based on its anatomical features [3]. In mainland China, oblique vaginal septum syndrome (OVSS) has been proposed as the Chinese nomenclature by Peking Union Medical College Hospital (PUMCH), which summarizes the anatomical features with simplicity. The pathogenesis of HWWS is still unclear. Several studies assume that the distal hypoplasia or dysplasia of the unilateral mesonephric duct leads to developmental failure of the ureteral

S. Song · N. Chen · L. Zhu (✉)
Department of Obstetrics and Gynecology, Peking Union Medical College Hospital, Peking Union Medical College, Chinese Academy of Medical Sciences, Beijing, China

L. Zhu et al. (eds.), *Diagnosis and Management of Female Obstructive Genital Malformations*, https://doi.org/10.1007/978-981-19-6759-7_8

bud and vagina of this side and affects the location and fusion of paramesonephric ducts, resulting in anatomical malformations of HWWS [4, 5].

8.1 Classification

Up to now, HWWS is usually classified into two types, the completely obstructed and incompletely obstructed. This classification system is only based on the severity of menstrual blood obstruction.

Complete and incomplete obstruction classification systems cannot precisely display the anatomical features of different types. Actually, HWWS with various anatomical variants can be observed in clinical practice [6]. PUMCH classified HWWS into three subtypes by different anatomical features in 1985 and extended this classification system into four subtypes in 2015 [7–9]. These four subtypes are HWWS with blind hemivagina, HWWS with partial reabsorption of vaginal septum, HWWS with communicating cervix, and HWWS with cervicovaginal atresia. Figure 8.1 illustrates the anatomical features of different subtypes.

HWWS with blind hemivagina (type 1): This type has a complete blind hemivagina, while the uterus behind the septum is completely isolated from the contralateral one. There is no communication between the affected and unaffected side, resulting in a hematocele behind the vaginal septum.

HWWS with partial reabsorption of vaginal septum (type 2): There are small holes on the vaginal septum. The uterus behind the septum is also isolated from the other one. Therefore, menstrual blood can flow out through the holes on the septum, but the drainage is impeded.

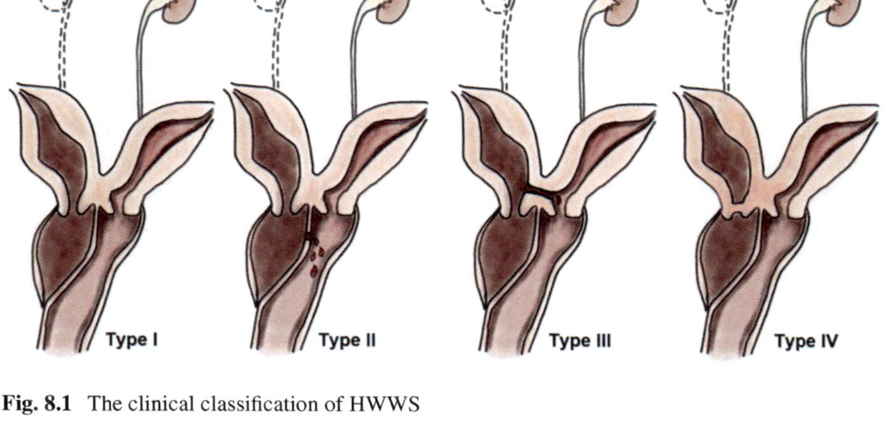

Fig. 8.1 The clinical classification of HWWS

HWWS with communicating uteri (type 3): This type has a complete blind hemivagina but a small fistula between cervices. The menstrual blood of the affected side can flow out through the contralateral uterus with limited drainage.
HWWS with cervical vaginal atresia (type 4): The cervix behind the vaginal septum is maldeveloped or atretic, resulting in hematometra of the affected side.

8.2 Clinical Manifestations

Symptoms of HWWS are mainly caused by poor menstrual blood drainage, secondary infection, and hematocele compression. Patients with complete obstruction subtype generally present with symptoms shortly after menarche, while patients with incomplete vaginal obstruction show symptoms significantly later [10]. Patients might present with the following symptoms.

Pain: Most patients display dysmenorrhea and periodic lower abdominal pain, especially in patients with type 1 and type 4 HWWS. A small fraction of patients might have chronic pelvic pain or dyspareunia.
Abnormal vaginal discharge: This symptom often arises in type 2 and type 3 HWWS patients. Abnormal vaginal discharge can be irregular vaginal hemorrhage or intermittent mucopurulent discharge.
Compression symptoms: Some patients might show frequent urination, dysuria, urinary retention, or tenesmus caused by hematocele compression.

8.3 Physical Examination

Doctors might observe a bulging vaginal septum in a HWWS patient with broad vaginal opening. This sign is common in type 1 HWWS patients. A cystic mass can be touched on the vaginal wall by bimanual examination. In addition, two uterine corpora can be touched, often along with the enlarged uterus of the affected side. If a patient is sexually inexperienced, doctors can perform recto-abdominal examination. Generally, a pelvic mass can be touched, with or without tenderness. The tenderness might be prominent when the mass is infected.

8.4 Complications and Fertility Outcome

The main complications of HWWS are endometriosis and infection. According to statistics, endometriosis occurs in about 20% of HWWS patients. This rate is significantly higher in patients with complete vaginal obstruction [11]. Patients with incomplete vaginal obstruction are susceptible to ascending infection. When patients present with abdominal pain and fever, doctors should screen for acute or chronic pelvic inflammation, such as pelvic abscess.

The fertility outcome is satisfactory in HWWS patients who received treatment timely. Candiani et al. performed a long-term follow-up in 36 HWWS cases postoperatively. The pregnancy rate was 87% and the live birth rate was 77% [12]. PUMCH also analyzed 70 postoperative patients in 2013 and found that the pregnancy rate was 84.8% [10].

8.5 Diagnosis

The diagnosis of HWWS should meet the anatomical features of uterine didelphys, obstructed hemivagina, and ipsilateral renal anomalies.

8.5.1 Diagnostic Methods

1. Pelvic and urinary system ultrasound: This is the first-line method because it is cost-effective and noninvasive. Pelvic ultrasound can observe uterine didelphys, hematocele, and secondary endometrial cysts or abscesses. Urinary system ultrasound can identify malformations such as renal agenesis, ectopic kidney, or duplex kidney.
2. Pelvic magnetic resonance imaging (MRI): Pelvic MRI is more accurate in identifying a specific clinical classification, complications, and complicated malformations, especially in diagnosing type 4 HWWS [13]. Figure 8.2 shows pelvic MRI images of HWWS patients.
3. Diagnostic vaginoscopy: Doctors could use diagnostic vaginoscopy to visualize the vaginal canal to avoid damaging the hymen and lower genital tract [14].

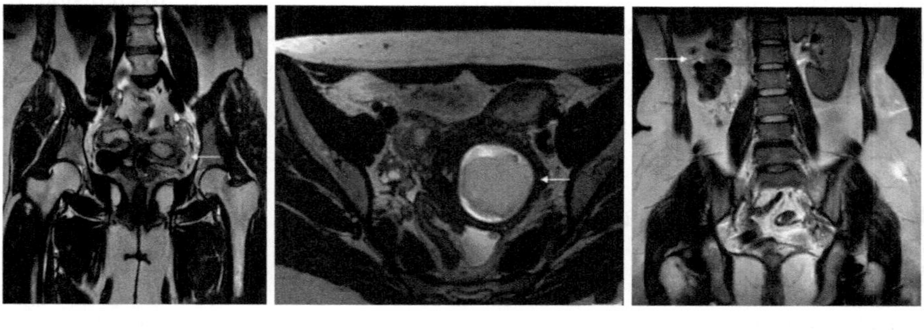

Fig. 8.2 Pelvic MRI of patients with HWWS. The arrow in (**a**) shows uterus didelphys. The arrow in (**b**) shows a huge hematocele behind the vaginal septum. The arrow in (**c**) shows the right renal agenesis in patients with HWWS

8.5.2 *Differential Diagnosis*

1. Vaginal cysts: Vaginal cysts appear as bulges in the vaginal wall without periodic change. Generally, patients will not present with periodic pelvic pain. Ultrasound will identify normal anatomy of uterus, bilateral adnexa, and urinary system.
2. Pelvic abscess: Patients always show fever with abdominal pain. Physical examination will not identify a bulge in the vaginal wall. Elevated white blood cell count and inflammatory indicators, pyosalpinx, or pelvic abscess observed in ultrasound or MRI will also support this diagnosis. However, ascending infection is a common complication of HWWS. Doctors should be alert to the possibility of HWWS complicated with pelvic abscess.
3. Ovarian mass: Patients might begin with abdominal pain and pelvic mass. Pelvic examination could identify a mass in a relatively high location and no bulge in vaginal wall. Pelvic ultrasound will observe mass in adnexa area. But doctors should rule out HWWS complicated with endometrial cysts during differential diagnosis.

8.6 Treatment

Surgery is the most effective treatment method to relieve obstruction, prevent complications, and preserve fertility. For patients with clinical symptoms after menarche, surgical treatment is recommended as soon as possible after definite diagnosis. However, there is little guidance on the management for prepubertal patients. Though it is reported that infants prior to 6 months of age might have vaginal distension due to maternal estrogen, most of them achieved complete resolution without treatment. The majority of HWWS cases diagnosed in prepuberty can be conservatively managed without need for vaginal surgery. Elective surgeries performed after menarche and before detecting complications could achieve higher success rate and lower recurrence rate [15, 16].

8.6.1 *Vaginal Septum Resection Under Direct Vision*

We recommend performing this surgery when the hematocele is relatively large, as a large distended hematocolpos is easy to visualize and locate. During surgery, we should puncture the hematocele with a needle from the most prominent part. Drainage of accumulated hematocele or pus indicates the location is satisfactory. After the successful location, the incision is extended with a sharp knife to resect as much of the vaginal septum as possible, therefore preventing readhesion postoperatively. Surgeons should place a metal catheter in the urethra and an index finger into the anus as a guide to avoid urethra/bladder or rectum damage.

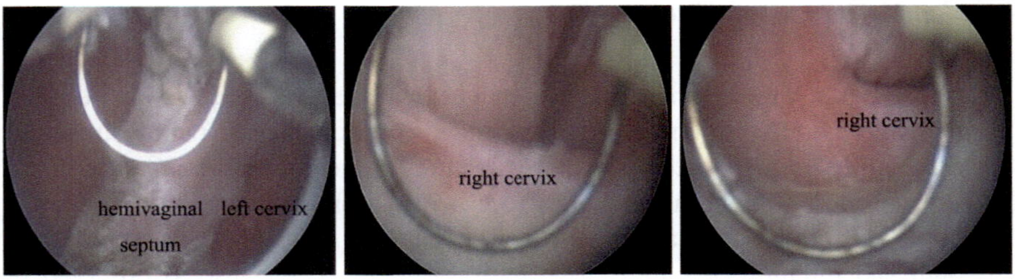

Fig. 8.3 Vaginal septum resection by vaginoscopy

8.6.2 Vaginal Septum Resection by Vaginoscopy

Vaginal septum resection by vaginoscopy or hysteroscopy could be a choice for patients who are sexually inexperienced and want to keep the hymen intact [17, 18]. Figure 8.3 shows pictures taken during the vaginal septum resection surgery by vaginoscopy.

8.6.3 Ipsilateral Hysterectomy

For patients with type 4 HWWS, it is recommended to perform ipsilateral hysterectomy. Surgeons should preserve as much uterine wall and cervix tissue of the unaffected side as possible during the operation.

8.7 Postoperative Management

The outcome is generally satisfactory in HWWS patients who have undergone timely operation. Patients should maintain regular follow-up for pelvic examination and ultrasound, in the case of postoperative readhesion. In addition, HWWS patients should monitor renal function regularly due to their renal anomalies.

References

1. Zhou Y, Fu X, Qian H, et al. A Herlyn-Werner-Wunderlich syndrome variant with ipsilateral renal absence and a contralateral duplex collecting system in a 26-year-old female. Gynecol Obstet Investig. 2014;77(2):137–40. https://doi.org/10.1159/000357446.
2. Shimizu M, Sakai S, Ohta K, Miyamoto M, Yachie A. Uterus didelphys with obstructed hemivagina and contralateral multicystic dysplastic kidney. CEN Case Rep. 2015;4(1):61–4. https://doi.org/10.1007/s13730-014-0139-9.

3. Piazza MJ, De Carvalho NS, Peixoto APL, Urbanetz AA. Uterus didelphys with obstructed hemivagina and ipsilateral renal agenesis (OHVIRA syndrome). JBRA Assist Reprod. 2015;19(4):259–62. https://doi.org/10.5935/1518-0557.20150049.
4. Acién P. Embryological observations on the female genital tract. Hum Reprod. 1992;7(4):437–45. https://doi.org/10.1093/oxfordjournals.humrep.a137666.
5. Sánchez-Ferrer ML, Acién MI, del Campo F, Mayol-Belda MJ, Acién P. Experimental contributions to the study of the embryology of the vagina. Hum Reprod. 2006;21(6):1623–8. https://doi.org/10.1093/humrep/del031.
6. Fedele L, Motta F, Frontino G, Restelli E, Bianchi S. Double uterus with obstructed hemivagina and ipsilateral renal agenesis: pelvic anatomic variants in 87 cases. Hum Reprod. 2013;28(6):1580–3. https://doi.org/10.1093/HUMREP/DET081.
7. Bian ML, Huang RL, Wu BZ, Lian LJ, Song HZ. Congenital oblique vaginal septum. Chin J Obstet Gynecol. 1985;20(02):85–8. http://rs.yiigle.com/CN112141198502/965258.htm. Accessed April 27, 2020
8. Zhu L, Chen N, Tong JL, Wang W, Zhang L, Lang JH. New classification of Herlyn-Werner-Wunderlich syndrome. Chin Med J. 2015;128(2):222–5. https://doi.org/10.4103/0366-6999.149208.
9. Chinese expert consensus on the diagnosis and treatment of obstructive uterine and vaginal dysplasia. Chin J Obstet Gynecol Pediatr 2021;56(11):746–52. https://doi.org/10.3760/CMA.J.CN112141-20210824-00466.
10. Tong J, Zhu L, Lang J. Clinical characteristics of 70 patients with Herlyn-Werner-Wunderlich syndrome. Int J Gynecol Obstet. 2013;121(2):173–5. https://doi.org/10.1016/j.ijgo.2012.11.023.
11. Tong J, Zhu L, Chen N, Lang J. Endometriosis in association with Herlyn-Werner-Wunderlich syndrome. Fertil Steril. 2014;102(3):790–4. https://doi.org/10.1016/j.fertnstert.2014.05.025.
12. Candiani GB, Fedele L, Candiani M. Double uterus, blind hemivagina, and ipsilateral renal agenesis: 36 cases and long-term follow-up. Obstet Gynecol. 1997;90(1):26–32. https://doi.org/10.1016/S0029-7844(97)83836-7.
13. Zhang J, Xu S, Yang L, Songhong Y. MRI image features and differential diagnoses of Herlyn–Werner–Wunderlich syndrome. Gynecol Endocrinol. Published online 2019. https://doi.org/10.1080/09513590.2019.1680623.
14. Fachin CG, Rocha JLAS, Maltoni AA, et al. Herlyn-Werner-Wunderlich syndrome: diagnosis and treatment of an atypical case and review of literature. Int J Surg Case Rep. 2019;63:129–34. https://doi.org/10.1016/J.IJSCR.2019.08.035.
15. Tan YG, Laksmi NK, Yap TL, Sadhana N, Ong CCP. Preventing the O in OHVIRA (obstructed hemivagina ipsilateral renal agenesis): early diagnosis and management of asymptomatic Herlyn-Werner-Wunderlich syndrome. J Pediatr Surg. Published online 2019. https://doi.org/10.1016/j.jpedsurg.2019.06.006.
16. Han JH, Lee YS, Im YJ, Kim SW, Lee M-J, Han SW. Clinical implications of obstructed hemivagina and ipsilateral renal anomaly (OHVIRA) syndrome in the prepubertal age group. PLoS One. 2016;11(11). https://doi.org/10.1371/JOURNAL.PONE.0166776.
17. Xu B, Xue M, Xu D. Hysteroscopic management of an oblique vaginal septum in a virgin girl with a rare variant of Herlyn-Werner-Wunderlich syndrome. J Minim Invasive Gynecol. 2015;22(1):7. https://doi.org/10.1016/J.JMIG.2014.08.002.
18. Zhang H, Pan H. Hysteroscopic management of an oblique vaginal septum with diverticulum in Herlyn-Werner-Wunderlich syndrome. J Minim Invasive Gynecol. 2021;28(9):1553–4. https://doi.org/10.1016/J.JMIG.2021.03.009.

Chapter 9
Transverse Vaginal Septum

Zichen Zhao, Shan Deng, and Lan Zhu

Abstract Transverse vaginal septum is a rare congenital malformation caused by incomplete canalization during embryonic development. It can be imperforate or perforated and cause obstructive or bleeding symptoms. Diagnosis can be made through physical examination, ultrasonography, and MRI. Complications include endometriosis, and the reproductive outcome needs further evaluation. Treatment involves surgical resection. Vaginal dilatation is performed in patients at high risk of vaginal stricture.

Keywords Transverse vaginal septum · Congenital malformation · Imperforate · Perforated · Management

The transverse vaginal septum is a rare malformation of the female genital tract, with an incidence from 1/84,000 to 1/2100 among women [1]. It is probably caused by incomplete canalization at the junction of the Müllerian duct and the urogenital sinus during embryonic development. Most patients present with a single septum located in the lower, middle, or upper part of the vagina (Fig. 9.1). Multiple septa can also be present occasionally [2, 3]. The thickness of the septum varies, usually thinner than 1 cm. The transverse vaginal septum can be divided into the imperforate and the perforated types (Fig. 9.2).

Z. Zhao · S. Deng · L. Zhu (✉)
Department of Obstetrics and Gynecology, Peking Union Medical College Hospital, Chinese Academy of Medical Sciences and Peking Union Medical College, Beijing, China

L. Zhu et al. (eds.), *Diagnosis and Management of Female Obstructive Genital Malformations*, https://doi.org/10.1007/978-981-19-6759-7_9

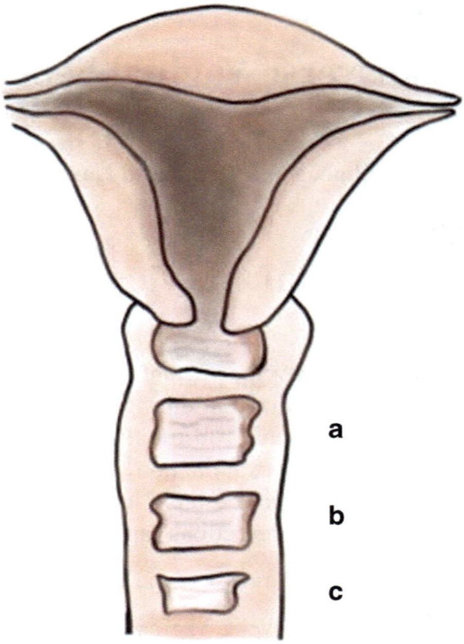

Fig. 9.1 The transverse vaginal septum with different locations. (**a**) Upper, (**b**) middle, and (**c**) lower septum

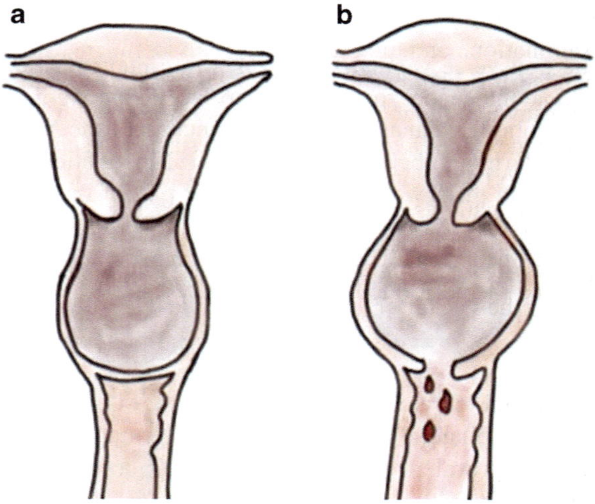

Fig. 9.2 The two types of transverse vaginal septum. (**a**) Imperforate septum and (**b**) perforated septum

9.1 Symptom

Due to the complete obstruction of the menstrual outflow tract, the patients with an imperforate septum, or obstructive septum, are associated with early onset of hematometra/hydrometra and hematocolpos/hydrocolpos during puberty, showing symptoms of primary amenorrhea, cyclic pain, dyspareunia, and primary infertility. Other symptoms caused by the compression of the resulting mass on surrounding organs include urinary frequency, dysuria, urinary retention, and feeling the need to defecate but unable to do so [4]. If there has been a spontaneous perforation in the septum, the patients may report sudden onset of heavy menstrual bleeding. An obstructive transverse vaginal septum is associated with mucus accumulation in the upper vagina in neonates and infants.

The perforated septum has a central or eccentric foramen that allows menstrual blood to flow out, leading to incomplete obstruction. The patients with perforated septum have irregular vaginal bleeding rather than obstructive symptoms [5] However, inadequate discharge of menstrual blood from micro-perforation may cause secondary infections, such as pyocolpos, pyometra, and some other pelvic inflammation [6].

The transverse vaginal septum is often comorbid with abnormalities of the urinary system, such as urethrovaginal fistulas, because differentiation of the urogenital sinus takes part in the formation of the bladder, urethra, and the vaginal vestibule [7]. If the partitioning of the cloaca into the urogenital sinus and anorectal canal goes wrong, rectal structural defects may occur, such as vaginal-rectal fistula, anal atresia, shared opening of the urogenital tract, and some other anomalies [8]. Besides, patients with transverse vaginal septum may also have a bicornuate uterus, aortic stenosis, atrial septal defect, and lumbar deformity [4].

9.2 Physical Examination

The patients with transverse vaginal septum have normal secondary sexual characteristics. The abdominal examination finds tenderness or abdominal mass in patients with an imperforate septum due to the hematometra/hydrometra and hematocolpos. Normal vulva and hymen are noted normal on inspection. The bimanual examination reveals a shortened vagina with a blind end, and the upper vagina is inaccessible without a palpable cervix. A mass in front of the rectum may be palpable on digital examination. A bulge protruding from the vagina is present in patients with a low vaginal septum, similar to the imperforate hymen, but they have a normal hymen and extra-hymen vagina.

In patients with a perforated transverse vaginal septum, an opening in the center of the septum can be seen on examination, which may be misjudged as dysplastic cervix by inexperienced doctors.

9.3 Complications and Reproductive Outcome

Due to the obstruction of menstrual blood outflow, the patients with transverse vaginal septum have an increased risk of endometriosis. The patients can conceive and give birth after transverse septum resection theoretically, but the reproductive outcome needs to be further evaluated by large-scale research [4]. Evidence showed that the pregnancy rate in low-level transverse vaginal septum was higher than in the middle- or high-level septum [9].

9.4 Diagnosis

The imperforate transverse vaginal septum is easier to diagnose than the perforated septum. The diagnosis should be considered in any patient with relevant clinical manifestations when an abdominal or pelvic mass is palpable or a shortened vagina with a blind end rather than a cervix is found on physical examination. The diagnosis is further confirmed by ultrasonography or magnetic resonance imaging (MRI).

The patients with perforated septum have atypical clinical manifestations, leading to a missed diagnosis. Patients with middle- or low-level transverse vaginal septum may have difficulty placing the tampons or having sexual intercourse. Thin and high-level septa are inefficiently detected by imaging inspection.

The common imaging methods are as follows:

1. Pelvic ultrasonography

   Pelvic ultrasonography is the initial diagnostic method for patients with cyclic pain, amenorrhea, or persistent pelvic pain. Cystic masses in the uterus and vagina can be seen in most patients with a transverse vaginal septum.
2. Pelvic MRI

   Pelvic MRI helps identify hematometra and hematocolpos and evaluates the location and thickness of the septum. It can clearly show the cervix, differentiating high-level transverse vaginal septum from cervical aplasia.

Transverse vaginal septum needs to be differentiated from other obstructive genital tract malformations such as cervical hypoplasia, vaginal atresia (referring to Chaps. 3 and 4), and imperforate hymen [4]. The presence of a bulge may occur in the cases of the low-level transverse vaginal septum, similar to that which happens in patients with imperforate hymen, but it does not move with Valsalva maneuvers [3].

9.5 Management

Vaginal septum excision should be performed to relieve the obstruction. Given the risk of retrograde infection, the puncture is not recommended for decompression of hematocolpos. The time of surgery is conroversial [10]. Most patients with imperforate septum show symptoms at puberty and should undergo surgery immediately after diagnosis. Although vaginal septum excision can relieve pain and reduce the risk of endometriosis, delayed surgery also has several advantages. Greater reproductive and psychological maturity at an elder age improves patients' compliance with vaginal dilation, and the production of estrogen after puberty promotes wound healing.

9.5.1 Menstrual Suppression

Menstrual suppression should be considered initially for adolescents who cannot cooperate with postoperative vaginal dilation. And the time of surgery should be delayed until the patients are psychologically prepared, understand the vaginal dilatation process, and can participate in joint decision-making. For inexperienced general medical centers, menstrual suppression can help improve patients' pain and provide time for referrals. Optional medications include oral contraceptives, highly effective progestin pills or injections, or GnRH-a [4].

9.5.2 Preoperative Preparation

Prophylactic antibiotics are recommended to be used. Bowel preparation contributes to rectal decompression, permitting a wider surgical field and minimizing incisional contamination. A Foley catheter is placed as a guide to avoid urethral injury during operation.

9.5.3 Surgical Process

The procedure to be performed depends on the thickness of the transverse vaginal septum. A cross incision is performed for the thin septum, and then the septum tissue is removed along the circumference of the vaginal wall. It is followed by end-to-end anastomosis of the upper and lower vaginal mucosa. It is more difficult to excise a thick transverse septum. A Foley catheter serves to locate the bladder and urethra, and a finger in the rectum helps avoid rectal injury. Due to the high risk of postoperative restenosis and obstruction, an experienced surgeon should perform the vaginal septum excision, or the patient should be referred to a center experienced in treating congenital female genital tract malformations, if necessary. Postoperatively, vaginal dilation should be carried out with a vaginal stent placed into the vagina [2].

Some other surgical procedures have been proposed, including Z-plasty (double cross) (Fig. 9.3) and Y-plasty (Fig. 9.4), based on staggered vaginal flaps [1, 11]. Covering the exposed vaginal wall with septum tissue may prevent the formation of circular scars and reduce the risk of postoperative vaginal stricture. In addition, as these plastic surgeries do not remove any tissue, vaginal shortening can be avoided.

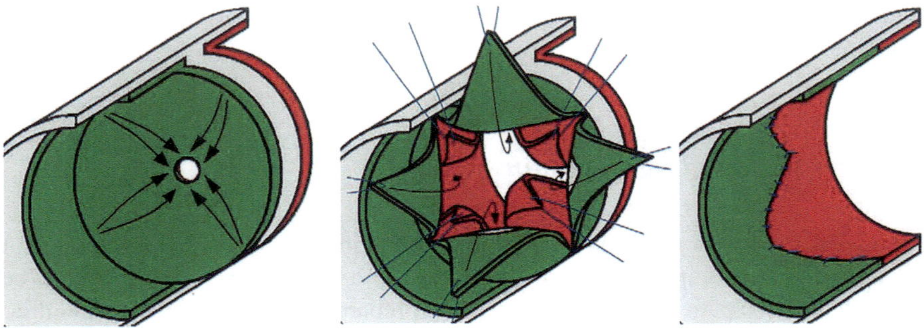

Fig. 9.3 Z-plasty of transverse vaginal septum. (Copy from Wierrani et al. [12])

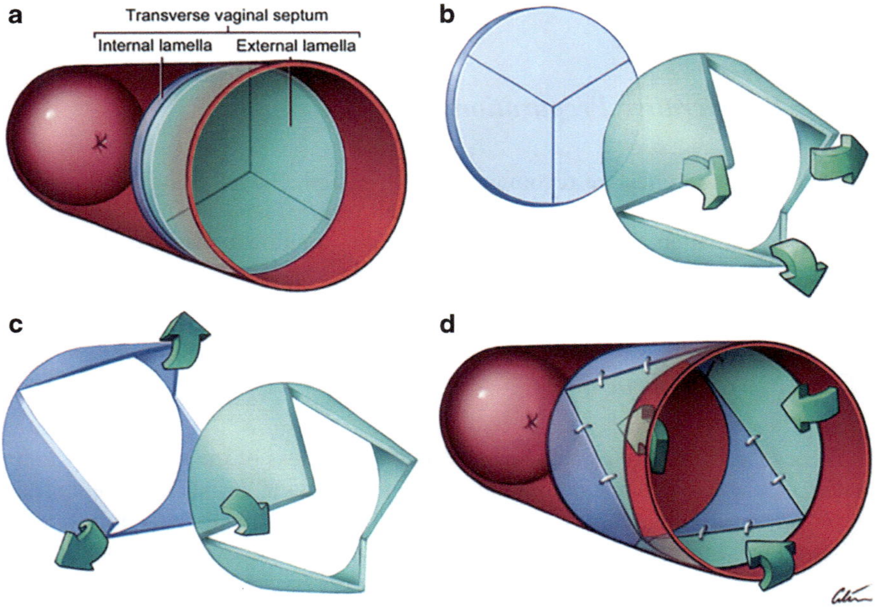

Fig. 9.4 Y-plasty. Demonstration of principle of Y-plasty technique. (**a**) Imperforate vaginal septum; note external and internal lamellae. Interstitial areolar tissue of variable thickness normally occupies interlamellar space. (**b**) Inverted Y-plasty on external lamella produces three external flaps; these will eventually be turned inward. (**c**) Y-plasty on internal lamella produces three internal flaps; these are turned outward. (**d**) External flaps are inverted and interdigitated with internal ones. Note the zigzag pattern of the resulting scar. (Copy from Arkoulis et al. [1])

The cruciate incision is made on the distal layer, and four flaps are made. The cruciform incision on the proximal layer is at a right angle to the previous incision on the distal flap. The apices joined to the basal intersection create a zigzag suture line.

9.5.4 Vaginal Dilation

There is controversy about the need for vaginal dilation before operation [11]. Some surgeons believe that preoperative vaginal dilation can be used to evaluate the patients' compliance, make the septum thinner, and expand the available vaginal tissue, which is beneficial to the anastomosis. Postoperative vaginal dilation is for patients who underwent laparoscopy or laparotomy and transvaginal surgery with a vaginal graft or obvious scar. And vaginal dilation should start as early as possible after the operation [2].

Patients who have undergone vaginoplasty, a thick vaginal septum removal, or skin flap transplantation have a higher risk of vaginal stricture. It is usually necessary to stay in bed with a vaginal stent in place for more than 7 days. A silicone vaginal stent or packed gauze may be used and covered with a sterile condom or glove. At the same time, a retaining urinary catheter, menstrual suppression, and deep venous thrombosis prophylaxis should be prescribed. After removing the vaginal stent, the patients should be instructed to stick to vaginal dilation until 3 months after surgery, to maintain the surgical effect [5].

9.5.5 Postoperative Complication

Acute postoperative complications include infection, intestinal or bladder injury, pain, and venous thromboembolism. Long-term complications include vaginal shortening, vaginal stricture, vaginal dilation pain, infertility, sexual difficulties, and psychological disorders. Postoperative vaginal stricture mostly occurs in patients who do not insist on vaginal dilation and need to dilate the vagina further. When the effect of dilation is unsatisfactory, additional surgical intervention is needed [11].

9.6 Postoperative Management

Following vaginal septum excision, the Foley catheter can be removed on the same day in patients with a low risk of vaginal stricture and resume their diet and daily activities under tolerable conditions. Regular vaginal dilation should be performed when necessary under guidance. Intercourse is forbidden for 6 weeks after surgery.

The patients should be reexamined after 3 months to ensure an unobstructed vagina [5].

References

1. Arkoulis N, Kearns C, Deeny M, Telfer J. The interdigitating Y-plasty procedure for the correction of transverse vaginal septa. BJOG. 2017;124:331–5.
2. Williams CE, Nakhal RS, Hall-Craggs MA, et al. Transverse vaginal septae: management and long-term outcomes. BJOG. 2014;121:1653–8.
3. Ziegler M, Azizkhan RG, von Allmen D, Weber TR. Operative Pediatric Surgery. New York: McGraw-Hill Education; 2014.
4. Management of acute obstructive uterovaginal anomalies: ACOG Committee Opinion, Number 779. Obstet Gynecol. 2019;133:e363–71.
5. Cetinkaya K, Kumtepe Y. Perforated transverse vaginal septum: a rare case of Müllerian duct anomaly presenting only primary infertility. Fertil Steril. 2008;90:2005.e11–3.
6. Schaffer JI, Hoffman BL, Bradshaw KD, Halvorson LM, Corton MM, Schorge JO. Williams gynecology. 4th ed. McGraw-Hill Education; 2020.
7. Amer MI, Ahmed Mel S, Ali AH. Congenital urethrovaginal fistula with transverse vaginal septum. J Obstet Gynaecol Res. 2016;42:1042–5.
8. Nathan L, Roman AS, Laufer N, DeCherney AH. Current diagnosis & treatment obstetrics & gynecology. 12th ed. New York: McGraw-Hill Education; 2019.
9. Rock JA, Zacur HA, Dlugi AM, Jones HW Jr, TeLinde RW. Pregnancy success following surgical correction of imperforate hymen and complete transverse vaginal septum. Obstet Gynecol. 1982;59:448–51.
10. Brander EPA, Vincent S, McQuillan SK. Transverse vaginal septum resection: technique, timing, and the utility of dilation. A scoping review of the literature. J Pediatr Adolesc Gynecol. 2022;35:65–72.
11. Sardesai SP, Dabade R, Chitale V. Double cross plasty for management of transverse vaginal septum: a 20-year retrospective review of our experience. J Obstet Gynaecol India. 2015;65:181–5.
12. Wierrani F, Bodner K, Spängler B, Grünberger W. "Z"-plasty of the transverse vaginal septum using Garcia's procedure and the Grünberger modification. Fertil Steril. 2003;79:608–12.

Part V
Obstructive Hymenal Malformations

Chapter 10
Congenital Hymen Abnormality

Ze Liang and Lan Zhu

Abstract The imperforate hymen is one of the most common congenital hymen abnormalities. As one of the obstructive female tract abnormalities, the typical manifestation is primary amenorrhea and periodic lower abdominal pain. Typically, no vaginal opening and mucosa with blue-purple cystic mass bulges within bilateral labial are found during physical examinations. Ultrasonography or MRI can help to differentially diagnose vaginal septum and vaginal atresia. The traditional surgical technique is to make a cross incision on the virginal membrane, remove multiple tissues, and suture the edge of the virginal membrane with absorbable suture.

Keywords Imperforate hymen · Hymenotomy · Lower genital tract obstruction

During neonatal development, when a layer of stratified squamous epithelium around the vaginal orifice does not spontaneously rupture, it is called virginal membrane dysplasia, which is shown in Fig. 10.1a–d. Among them, the most common is membranous atresia, which can be further divided into complete obstruction and incomplete obstruction [1].

Z. Liang · L. Zhu (✉)
Department of Obstetrics and Gynecology, Peking Union Medical College Hospital, Peking Union Medical College, Chinese Academy of Medical Sciences, Beijing, China

L. Zhu et al. (eds.), *Diagnosis and Management of Female Obstructive Genital Malformations*, https://doi.org/10.1007/978-981-19-6759-7_10

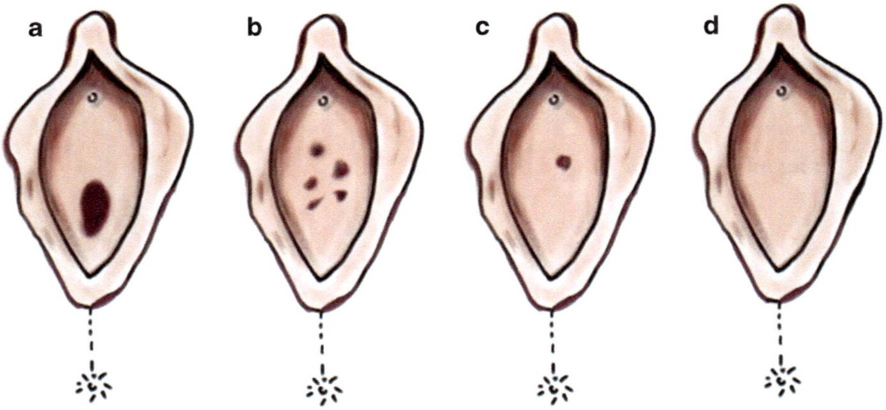

Fig. 10.1 Schematic drawing of different types of imperforate hymen. (**a**) Normal hymen. (**b**) Membranes imperforate hymen. (**c**) Microperforate hymen. (**d**) Complete imperforate hymen

10.1 Imperforate Hymen

The imperforate hymen is one of the rare causes of primary amenorrhea, which can cause female genital and urinary tract obstruction in the perinatal period, childhood, or adolescence. Infants with imperforate hymen may produce mucinous cysts due to endogenous maternal estrogen stimulation [2].

10.1.1 Symptoms

The clinical manifestations of imperforate hymen are diverse, depending on the age of onset, the severity of obstruction, and clinical course. Careful evaluation and differential diagnosis should be performed when dealing with infants or adolescent women, respectively. Female genital abnormalities may be difficult to identify in neonatal physical examination due to excessive tissue in virgin membranes. Due to endogenous maternal estrogen stimulation, infants may have vaginal mucus accumulation from vaginal and cervical gland secretion accumulation. Early pediatric manifestations may include urinary retention or hydronephrosis with urinary tract infection, and even acute kidney disease due to urinary tract obstruction [3].

Clarifying the history of menstruation is the most important issue when collecting the history of adolescent patients. Periodic pain is often caused by menstrual blood within the vagina and uterine bleeding. Obstruction can cause many pelvic

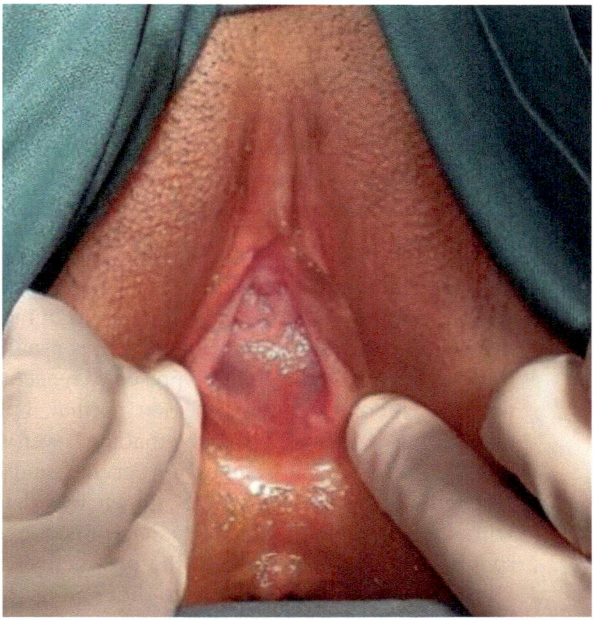

Fig. 10.2 Typical presentation of complete imperforate hymen

symptoms, including pelvic and back pain, constipation, sacral plexus irritation secondary to radiation pain, and urinary retention.

10.1.2 Physical Examinations

Female genital examination should start from the observation of the vulva. Typically, no vaginal opening and mucosa with blue-purple cystic mass bulges within bilateral labial are found during physical examinations (Fig. 10.2).

10.1.3 Diagnostic Criteria

Adolescent patients had periodic abdominal pain and no menstrual cramps. Gynecological examination showed that there was no vaginal opening in the vulva, and the perineal mucosa was a purple-blue protrusion. A cystic solid mass could be touched above the finger through rectal-abdominal examination. Ultrasound examination helps to determine the location and thickness of the septum and the distance from the obstructive tissue to the vaginal orifice. Ultrasonography or MRI can help to differentially diagnose vaginal septum and vaginal atresia.

10.2 Differential Diagnosis

1. The differential diagnosis of neonatal perineal mass includes periurethral cyst and ectopic ureter cyst prolapse. In either case, urethral and vaginal openings can be seen around the urethral cyst. Ectopic ureter cysts can be removed from the urethra and have a congested appearance.
2. Other vaginal abnormalities caused by abnormal development of urogenital tract and Müllerian duct are:

   (a) Vaginal septum: Vaginal septum can be located at different levels (upper, middle, and lower) in the vagina. The virgin membrane is often visible and normal. The thickness of the diaphragm is usually less than 1 cm, and a central or eccentric hole might be present. Gynecological examination showed that the external genitalia seemed normal, but bimanual examination or endoscopic examination showed that the lower vaginal segment was shorter, and the upper vaginal segment or cervix could not be seen. Masses can be touched above the inspection finger by rectal-abdominal examination. Ultrasound examination helps to determine the location and thickness of the septum and the distance from the obstructive tissue to the vaginal orifice. Ultrasonography or MRI helps to differentiate high transverse septum from congenital absence of cervix.

   (b) Vaginal atresia: Vaginal atresia is a reproductive tract obstructive disease, which is commonly found at puberty. It is mainly manifested as primary amenorrhea with periodic lower abdominal pain. Patients with type I vaginal atresia had normal uterus and endometrial function, accompanied by early and severe symptoms. During the examination, the location of the pelvic mass was relatively low, which was mostly located in front of the rectum. The development of the uterus and endometrial function in patients with type II vaginal atresia was slightly poor, and the symptoms appeared late and mild. As a result, the treatment time was relatively late. Due to the expansion of the upper vaginal segment or uterine cavity of the patient due to blood retention, pelvic masses can be touched when gynecological examination is performed in double or triple combination. Pelvic ultrasonography and/or pelvic magnetic resonance imaging can identify the presence of upper vaginal and/or uterine bleeding (or effusion), which is helpful for the diagnosis of vaginal atresia.

10.2.1 Treatment

It has been reported that spontaneous rupture of the hymen may occur in infants with asymptomatic hymen atresia of 1 day or 1 month old. Imperforate hymen can be found in neonatal physical examination, when abdominal pain symptoms can be emergency treatment. Hymenotomy should be performed under general anesthesia [4].

The traditional method of excision of the virginal membrane is to make a cross incision on the virginal membrane, remove multiple tissues in each quadrant, and suture the edge of the virginal membrane with absorbable suture. It is not recommended to puncture and drain. Re-atresia of the hymen may be related to ascending infection and reproductive complications. A study using a laser to create new holes under local anesthesia was conducted on 13 patients aged 12–16. The patients were followed up for 2 weeks without scars or stenosis, and no rejection response without applying estrogen cream at 18 months.

10.2.2 Postoperative Management and Prognosis

Surgical patients have good prognosis. Adolescents with surgical treatment have few sexual difficulties in adulthood. Long-term follow-up of 40 patients with virginal atresia found that the success rate of full-term pregnancy in patients with virginal atresia was significantly better [5].

References

1. Kimberley N, Hutson JM, Southwell BR, Grover SR. Vaginal agenesis, the hymen, and associated anomalies. J Pediatr Adolesc Gynecol. 2012;25(1):54–8. https://doi.org/10.1016/j.jpag.2011.08.003.
2. Laghzaoui O. Congenital imperforate hymen. 2016: 1–2. https://doi.org/10.1136/bcr-2016-215124.
3. Lee KH et al. Imperforate hymen: a comprehensive systematic review. J Clin Med. https://doi.org/10.3390/jcm8010056.
4. Miller RJ, Breech LL. Surgical correction of vaginal anomalies. Clin Obstet Gynecol. 2008;51(2):223–36.
5. Deligeoroglou E, Deliveliotou A, Makrakis E, Creatsas G. Concurrent imperforate hymen, transverse vaginal septum, and unicornuate uterus: a case report. J Pediatr Surg. 2007:1446–8. https://doi.org/10.1016/j.jpedsurg.2007.03.067.

Part VI
Obstructive Cloacal Malformations

Chapter 11
Cloacal Malformations

Jiali Duan and Lan Zhu

Abstract Cloacal malformations (CM), also called persistent cloaca (PC) or partial urorectal septum malformation (pURSM), are characterized by the confluence of the urethra, vagina, and rectum into one common channel (CC), which is identified on the perineum as a single orifice (Fig. 11.1). Occurring only in women, CM is the most complex type of anorectal malformations (ARM) with large anatomical variation among patients [1]. The incidence was estimated to be about 1 in 50,000 newborn girls, causing limited experience in diagnosis and treatment [2, 3]. The pathogenesis remains largely unknown, which may be related to the abnormal development of the urorectal septum during the embryonic stage. CM affects the urinary system, digestive system, and female reproductive system at the same time. The operation aims to restore the normal anatomy and function of the urethra, vagina, and rectum, which is complicated and requires long-term follow-up with multidisciplinary cooperation. This section focuses on the reproductive tract obstruction caused by CM combined with Müllerian duct system malformation.

Keywords Cloacal malformations · Persistent cloaca · Partial urorectal septum malformation · Anorectal malformations

---

J. Duan · L. Zhu (✉)
Department of Obstetrics and Gynecology, Peking Union Medical College Hospital, Peking Union Medical College, Chinese Academy of Medical Sciences, Beijing, China

L. Zhu et al. (eds.), *Diagnosis and Management of Female Obstructive Genital Malformations*, https://doi.org/10.1007/978-981-19-6759-7_11

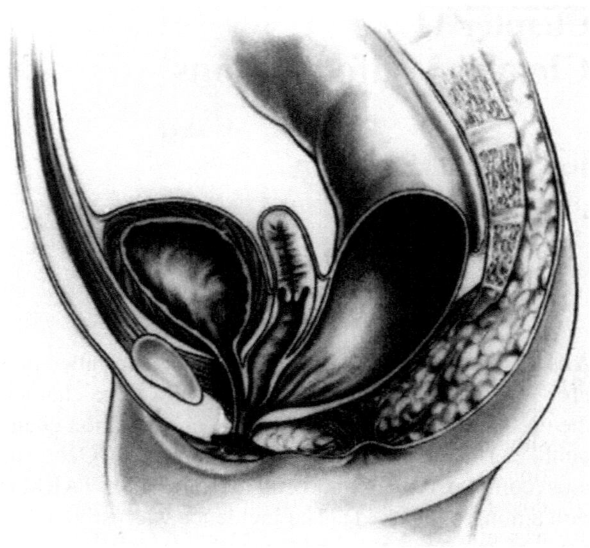

Fig. 11.1 Schematic diagram showing the anatomy of cloacal malformations. (From [4])

11.1 Symptoms and Signs

CM is often diagnosed during the physical examination of the newborn when there is no opening in the normal anal position, and only one single opening in the perineum is found (Fig. 11.2.).

Gynecological manifestations at different growth stages are as follows:

1. Infancy: About 30–40% of CM patients have hydrocolpos (Fig. 11.3) [5], and a mass in the lower abdomen can be palpated, which is more common when the common duct is long or when the two vaginas are combined [6]. If the effusion is not treated in time, on the one hand, it may progress to vaginal empyema, vaginal fibrosis, etc., which will bring difficulties to vaginoplasty; on the other hand, fluid pressure on the bladder triangle can lead to water accumulation in the bladder, hydroureter, hydronephrosis, and even renal failure [7].

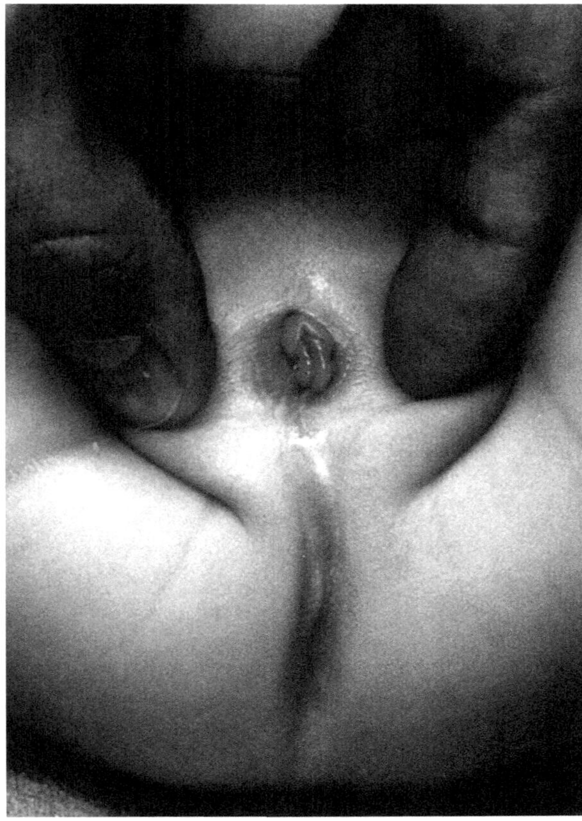

Fig. 11.2 Pictures showing the single opening in the perineum of CM patients. (From [4])

2. Adolescence: Approximately 40 percent of CM patients present with lower abdominal pain due to obstructed menstrual flow; about 20% of CM patients present with primary amenorrhea [6].
3. Adulthood: About half of the patients presented with dyspareunia due to vaginal retraction and stricture, requiring another vaginoplasty [8].

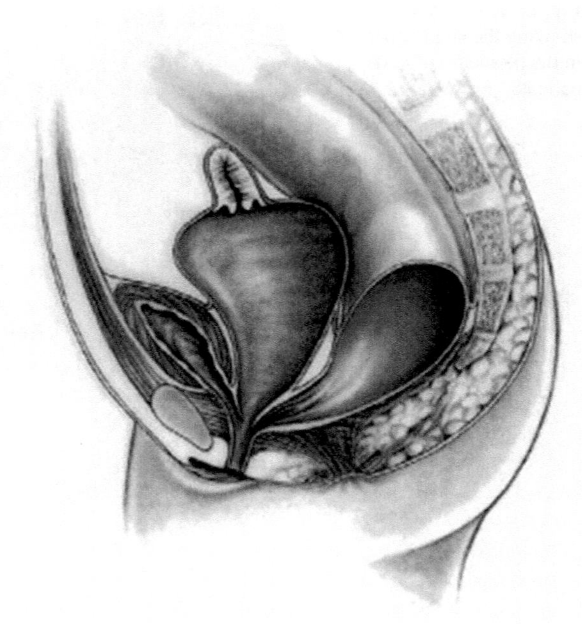

Fig. 11.3 Schematic diagram showing the anatomy of CM with hydrocolpos. (From [4])

11.2 Complications and Pregnancy Outcomes

About 50% of CM patients, especially when the common duct length is larger than 3 cm, have Müllerian duct malformation, manifested as uterine didelphys, longitudinal vaginal septum, bicornuate uterus, vaginal septum, etc [6] Concurrent malformations include vertebral-anorectal-cardiac-tracheoesophageal-renal-limb (VACTERL) syndrome, tethered spinal cord, and sacral dysplasia.

Pregnancy outcomes of CM patients are strongly related to comorbid genital tract malformations: if the patient has no uterus, she cannot conceive; if the patient has a unicornuate uterus, bicornuate uterus, or uterine didelphys, there is a higher risk of miscarriage and preterm birth [9]. Sanchez et al. summarized 13 patients with CM whose pregnancy outcomes were reported in the literature: most patients could conceive naturally, but the incidence of preterm birth, premature rupture of membranes, and cesarean section (12/13) was high [10]. Considering that most CM patients have concurrent malformations and the possibility of pelvic adhesions, the difficulty of cesarean section increases [10].

11.3 Diagnosis and Evaluation

11.3.1 Diagnostic Criteria and Classification

The diagnosis could be made by a physical examination which reveals only a single opening in the perineum.

Because infant girls' urethra and vaginal opening are not easy to expose, CM is often misdiagnosed as a congenital absence of anus with a rectovaginal fistula. As a result, the surgery includes anoplasty and the treatment of a rectovaginal fistula, leaving urogenital sinus problems untreated [4]. Therefore, a thorough physical examination should be performed at the initial diagnosis. If necessary, a suspicious perineal opening can be intubated to determine the direction of the fistula. Doctors should combine auxiliary examinations to avoid misdiagnosis, which leads to the failure of radical resection.

According to the length of the common channel (CC), CM is divided into two types by Pena classification [11]: (1) CC <3 cm type (short common channel type); (2) CC >3 cm type (long common channel type). The length of the CC affects the choice of surgical method and prognosis.

11.3.2 Initial Assessment

For newly diagnosed CM newborns, the goal of the initial assessment is to identify the presence of life-threatening deformities [4]:

1. Determine whether there is hydrocolpos or hydronephrosis through abdominal and pelvic ultrasound.
2. Confirm whether there is cardiac malformation by ECHO.
3. Determine whether there is spinal deformity through plain X-ray films of the lumbar spine and sacrum.
4. Determine whether there is a tethered spinal cord by spinal ultrasound.

11.3.3 Preoperative Assessment

The preoperative assessment aims to determine the length of the common channel, the length of the urethra, the location of the distal rectum, and the anatomy of the vagina to determine the surgical approach. Common auxiliary examinations include:

1. X-ray: Traditional inverted and lateral X-rays can only show the position of the end of the rectum without enough information about the urethra and vagina. Distal colonography and cloacography (common angiography) through the fistula are traditional methods that can dynamically display the channels [1].

Rotational fluoroscopy and three-dimensional reconstruction techniques developed in recent years can display the length of the common channel and the spatial relationship of the three channels. Still, children patients need general anesthesia and will be exposed to higher radiation doses [12].
2. Cysto-vaginoscopy can show the fine anatomical structures under direct vision, confirming the length of the urethra, the starting point, endpoint, and length of the common channel. All CM patients should undergo colposcopy to provide as much anatomical information of the reproductive tract as possible in order to plan proper treatment prior to menarche [6].
3. MRI: It has a high resolution on soft tissue, can provide spatial information on pelvic organs, and is suitable for evaluating the location of the distal end of the rectum and the length of the rectal fistula. However, the accuracy of measuring the length of the urethra and the common channel is limited. Therefore, MRI combined with cystoscopy is ideal for preoperative evaluation [1].

CM patients often have concurrent malformations, so the whole body should be systematically assessed during the preoperative assessment.

11.3.4 Evaluation of the Patency of the Müllerian System [6]

Reproductive tract patency examination before menarche can avoid the occurrence of menstrual obstruction. (1) Check whether there is mucus in the outer area of the cervix through colposcopy. If there is any, the cervix is unobstructed (Fig. 11.4). (2) Perform anterograde tubal perfusion during abdominal surgery to see whether saline

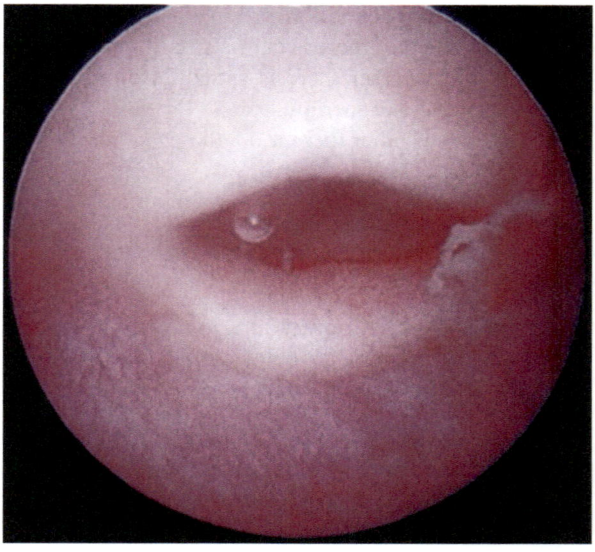

Fig. 11.4 The presence of mucus in the ectocervix. (From [6])

can flow out of the vaginal orifice. Suppose there is no opportunity to perform the above examinations before menarche. In that case, an ultrasound examination should be performed every 6–9 months after the breast development of CM children in order to monitor the presence of hematometra and hematocolpos. For adult patients, hysterosalpingography could be considered.

11.3.5 Prenatal Diagnosis

Prenatal diagnosis of CM is difficult. Prenatal three-dimensional ultrasonography and prenatal MRI can indicate anatomical deformities. Vaginal effusion is the most common prenatal sign of CM [13]. Prenatal ultrasound signs of suspected CM include cystic mass in the pelvis, vesicoureteral dilatation, and abnormal bowel dilation [14].

11.4 Treatment

CM patients require surgical treatment to correct anatomical deformities and restore physiological function. Considering the complexity of radical surgery and also that the genital systems of newborn patients are not fully developed, surgical treatment is usually carried out in two steps:

1. Palliative surgery: Within 24 h after birth, if hydrocolpos causes no acute lower urinary tract obstruction, palliative colostomy should be performed to solve the defecation problem. If the patient has hydrocolpos combined with uroschesis, vesicoureteral reflux, or ureterectasis, vaginal colostomy should be performed to drain fluid and relieve bladder outlet obstruction. If the patient has dual vaginas, a mediastinal window should be created to ensure adequate fluid drainage on both sides and avoid injury to the cervix [6].
2. Radical surgery: Radical surgery is usually performed 6–12 months after birth [4]. Radical resection consists of (1) separation and reconstruction of the posterior rectum and urogenital tract. If the end of the rectum is above the pubococcygeal line, posterior sagittal anorectoplasty (PSARP) can be performed. Otherwise, transabdominal surgery is needed (2) Separation and reconstruction of the anterior urethra and vagina. If the common channel's length is less than 3 cm and the length of the urethra is more than 1.5 cm, total urogenital mobilization (TUM) is preferred. The operation is relatively simple, with few complications and a good prognosis. Otherwise, the long common channel and short urethra may bring excessive dissociation resulting in failure of functional restoration, such as urinary incontinence and vaginal ischemic stenosis. In this situation, urogenital separation is required. The surgical plan is complicated with numerous complications and a relatively poor prognosis [4, 15].

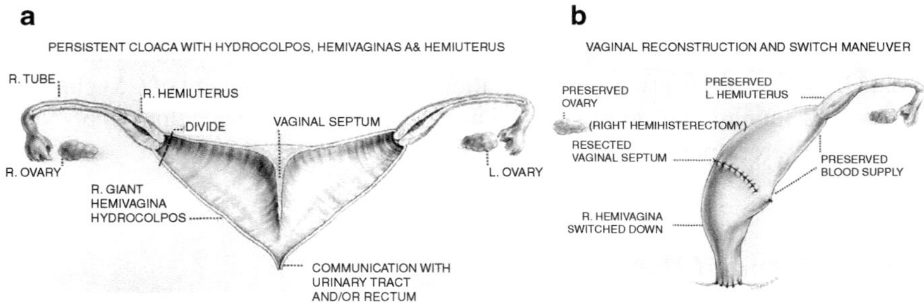

Fig. 11.5 Schematic diagram showing vaginal switch maneuver. (From [11]). (a) Two large dilated hemivaginas, two hemiuterus, and long common channel. (b) The right hemiuterus was resected with the right ovary reserved. The right hemivagina was switched down

The separation and reconstruction of the vagina is the most critical and complicated part of the operation [11]: If the common channel is short, vaginal pull-through can be performed. If there is a double uterus and double vagina, a vaginal switch maneuver can be considered (Fig. 11.5) [4]. If the patient has a short vagina that cannot be pulled to the perineum, a vaginal replacement procedure is needed. The vaginal reconstruction material can be selected from the rectum, small intestine, colon, buccal mucosa, etc. If the patient has a vaginal mediastinum, it should be removed during vaginal reconstruction [6]. As for the timing of surgery, vaginoplasty is currently performed at the same time as radical surgery. About 56% of patients require a second operation due to dyspareunia. Therefore, some views suggest that for CM patients without vaginal effusion, vaginoplasty can be postponed to before puberty. By combining vaginal dilation, the incidence of vaginal restenosis can be reduced, and the second operation can be reduced [9].

11.5 Postoperative Management

After radical resection, more than half of the patients can achieve voluntary control of urination and defecation through postoperative training [4].

With the improvement of surgical techniques, more and more CM patients can survive to adulthood. Therefore, the importance of regular obstetrics and gynecology follow-up is recognized.

1. Adolescence: Since it is difficult to clearly diagnose genital tract malformations in infancy [16], special attention should be paid to whether there are menarche and periodic lower abdominal pain after breast development begins. It would be better to monitor by ultrasound if permitted. If hematometra or hematocolpos is found, hormone suppression therapy should be administered immediately to avoid further accumulation of menstrual blood; and elective surgery should be performed to relieve the obstruction [6].

2. Adulthood: Patients should undergo a comprehensive gynecological examination before they have sexual needs to assess whether there is vaginal contracture and stenosis to ensure normal sexual function.
3. Before pregnancy: CM patients often have concurrent malformations. Therefore, when preparing for pregnancy, CM patients should discuss with an obstetrician to assess whether they can tolerate pregnancy and prepare in advance for possible premature birth, cesarean section, etc.

References

1. Versteegh HP, Gardner DS, Scriven L, et al. Reconsidering diagnosis, treatment, and postoperative care in children with cloacal malformations. J Pediatr Adolesc Gynecol. 2021;34(6):773–9.
2. Tennant PW, Glinianaia SV, Wellesley D, et al. Epidemiology of partial urorectal septum malformation sequence (or 'persistent cloaca'): a population-based study in seven regions of England and Wales, 1985–2010. Arch Dis Child Fetal Neonatal Ed. 2014;99(5):F413–8.
3. Halleran DR, Wood RJ. Cloacal Malformations. In: StatPearls. Treasure Island: StatPearls Publishing; 2022. Copyright © 2022, StatPearls Publishing LLC.
4. Peña A, Levitt M. Surgical management of cloacal malformations. Semin Neonatol. 2003;8(3):249–57.
5. Levitt MA, Pena A. Cloacal malformations: lessons learned from 490 cases. Semin Pediatr Surg. 2010;19(2):128–38.
6. Breech L. Gynecologic concerns in patients with cloacal anomaly. Semin Pediatr Surg. 2016;25(2):90–5.
7. Bischoff A, Levitt MA, Breech L, et al. Hydrocolpos in cloacal malformations. J Pediatr Surg. 2010;45(6):1241–5.
8. Couchman A, Creighton SM, Wood D. Adolescent and adult outcomes in women following childhood vaginal reconstruction for cloacal anomaly. J Urol. 2015;193(5 Suppl):1819–22.
9. Fernando MA, Creighton SM, Wood D. The long-term management and outcomes of cloacal anomalies. Pediatr Nephrol. 2015;30(5):759–65.
10. Vilanova-Sanchez A, Mccracken K, Halleran DR, et al. Obstetrical outcomes in adult patients born with complex anorectal malformations and cloacal anomalies: a literature review. J Pediatr Adolesc Gynecol. 2019;32(1):7–14.
11. Pena A, Levitt MA, Hong A, et al. Surgical management of cloacal malformations: a review of 339 patients. J Pediatr Surg. 2004;39(3):470–9; discussion 9.
12. Reck-Burneo CA, Lane V, Bates DG, et al. The use of rotational fluoroscopy and 3-D reconstruction in the diagnosis and surgical planning for complex cloacal malformations. J Pediatr Surg. 2019;54(8):1590–4.
13. Bischoff A, Levitt MA, Lim FY, et al. Prenatal diagnosis of cloacal malformations. Pediatr Surg Int. 2010;26(11):1071–5.
14. Livingston JC, Elicevik M, Breech L, et al. Persistent cloaca: a 10-year review of prenatal diagnosis. J Ultrasound Med. 2012;31(3):403–7.
15. Wood RJ, Reck-Burneo CA, Levitt MA. Cloacal malformations: technical aspects of the reconstruction and factors which predict surgical complexity. Front Pediatr. 2019;7:240.
16. Management of acute obstructive uterovaginal anomalies: ACOG Committee Opinion, Number 779. Obstet Gynecol. 2019;133(6):e363–71.

Chapter 12
Urogenital Sinus Malformations

Qianqian Gao, Jianbin Guo, Ze Liang, and Lan Zhu

Abstract Urogenital sinus (UGS) malformations are defined by the confluence of the urethra and vagina to form a common channel of varying length with a single perineal opening. The embryogenesis of UGS malformations was considered as the cessation of Müllerian ducts development at embryo ninth week. The clinical symptoms vary with the size of the urogenital sinus opening and the position of the urethral orifice; thus, the management should be individualized.

Keywords Urogenital sinus · Posterior cloaca · Genitalia

12.1 Definition

Urogenital sinus (UGS) malformations, also called common urogenital orifice, are defined by the confluence of the urethra and vagina to form a common channel of varying length with a single perineal opening. In this condition, the anorectal canal opens separately on the perineum. Peña et al. used the term "posterior cloaca" to describe this rare malformation [1]. According to the length of urogenital sinus and the position of urethral orifice, urogenital sinus malformations are divided into three subtypes (Fig. 12.1).

Q. Gao · J. Guo · Z. Liang · L. Zhu (✉)
Department of Obstetrics and Gynecology, Peking Union Medical College Hospital, Peking Union Medical College, Chinese Academy of Medical Sciences, Beijing, China

L. Zhu et al. (eds.), *Diagnosis and Management of Female Obstructive Genital Malformations*, https://doi.org/10.1007/978-981-19-6759-7_12

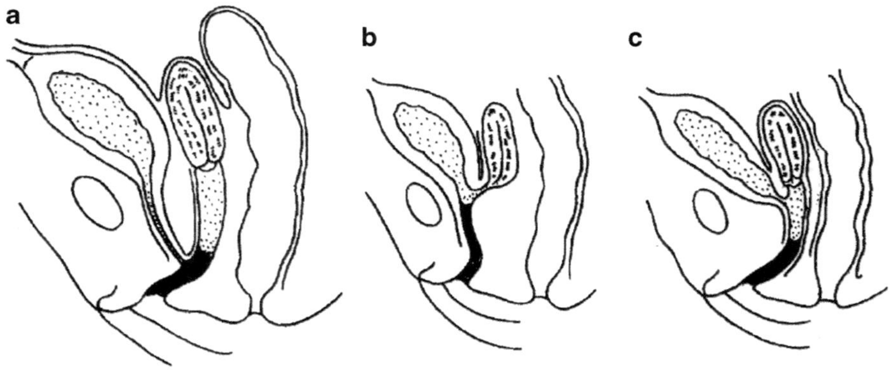

Fig. 12.1 Three subtypes of urogenital sinus malformations

12.2 Pathogenesis

At the end of the third week, the terminal hindgut dilates and communicates with the allantoic sac to form a cloaca. At the fourth week, the mesodermal folds between the cloaca and the hindgut grow caudally to form the urorectal septum, which divides the cloaca into urogenital sinus and rectum. In female embryos, the bilateral Müllerian ducts fuse at midline and extend caudally into the urorectal septum, dividing the urogenital sinus into urethral part and vaginal part [2]. During the embryo's ninth week, urogenital sinus malformations may occur if the development of Müllerian ducts ceases. The length of the common channel will be long if the development of Müllerian ducts stopped early, otherwise the length of the common channel will be short.

12.3 Clinical Manifestation

12.3.1 Symptoms

Clinical symptoms vary with the size of urogenital sinus opening and the position of urethral orifice. Patients with large sinus opening and low urethral orifice are usually asymptomatic or vulnerable to urinary tract infection. Urinary incontinence and periodic hematuria may occur in patients with high urethral orifice. The small sinus opening may be mistaken for the urethral opening; thus, patients will be misdiagnosed as congenital absence of vagina. These patients may suffer from dyspareunia. Patients with urogenital sinus malformations usually present with ambiguous external genitalia and often accompanied with duplication of uterus and vagina and anomalies of urinary system [3, 4].

12.3.2 Physical Examination

There is only one orifice in the perineum vestibular area, while the anorectal opening is normal.

12.4 Diagnosis

Clinical manifestations, laboratory tests, and imaging examinations are necessary for the diagnosis (Fig. 12.2).

1. Physical examination suggests there is only one orifice in the perineum vestibular area.

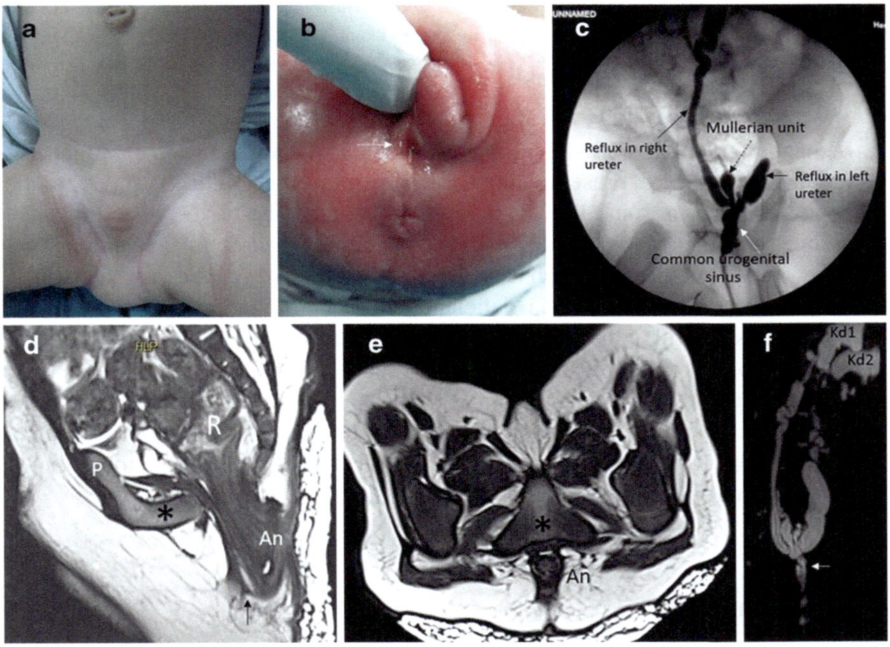

Fig. 12.2 Perineal development and imaging findings of urogenital sinus malformations. (From Abouzeid et al [4]). (**a**) "Doll-like" perineum. (**b**) A common urogenital orifice (white arrow) is markedly deviated posteriorly to open in the perineum slightly anterior to the anus. (**c**) Contrast X-ray study (genitogram) demonstrating a common urogenital sinus with reflux of contrast into both ureters and Müllerian structure; note the absence of urinary bladder. (**d** and **e**) Pelvic MRI (midsagittal and axial, respectively) demonstrating the exaggerated midline bony fusion of the pubis (P) and ischial bones (∗); the rectum (R) and anal canal (An) exit the pelvis behind the fused ischial tuberosities (∗). The black arrow in (**d**) points to the common urogenital orifice immediately in front of the anus. (**f**) Magnetic resonance urology (MRU) showing crossed fused renal ectopia; compare with genitogram in (**c**)

Patients present with 46, XX karyotype and normal female sex hormones.

2. Imaging examinations.

Pelvic ultrasound examination can help to show the female internal genitalia (uterus and ovaries).

Magnetic resonance imaging (MRI) can assess the confluence of the urethra and vagina and measure the length of the common channel accurately, which is of great value in exploring concomitant abnormalities of other organs (such as urinary tract abnormalities) and preoperative evaluation and surgical planning.

Cystourethroscopy and retrograde urography make it more accurate and visualized to detect the crucial and elaborate anatomical features, such as the length of common channel, confluence position of vagina and urethra and its adjacent relationship with bladder neck, development of vagina, presence of cervix, and anatomy of bladder and urethra, which is of great significance to evaluate the effect of reconstructive surgery [5].

12.5 Differential Diagnosis

1. Female pseudohermaphroditism: It can be manifested as the fusion of vagina and urethra. It is a typical presentation that hypertrophy of the clitoris is similar to the penis. The chromosome karyotype is 46XX. After puberty, there are laryngeal nodules and an obvious beard in patients. Most of the causes are congenital adrenal cortical hyperplasia, which is an autosomal recessive genetic disease, such as CYP21 deficiency and CYP11 deficiency. The determination of adrenocortical hormone is helpful to distinguish. A small part of the causes is that the mother is exposed to androgens during pregnancy, such as androgen-secreting tumors or taking exogenous androgens.
2. Labia minora fusion: It mostly occurs in prepuberty or postmenopausal women, which is related to low estrogen status. It is effective after menstruation or estrogen treatment.

12.6 Treatment

Individualized management shall be carried out according to the degree of defects. There are often no clinical symptoms or mild symptoms in patients with short common channel. In those patients, the opening of urethra and vagina is lower. Surgical interventions can be postponed until sex begins. For patients with longer common channels, urinary incontinence is often significant due to higher openings of urethra and vagina. The surgery is generally performed earlier.

The operations include clitoroplasty, labia reconstruction, and vaginoplasty. For cases with urinary incontinence, it is necessary to reconstruct the urethra with part of the vaginal wall. Children with kidney and urinary diseases are prone to early intervention. The cooperation of pediatrics, nephrology, and urology is helpful for the treatment of children. Preoperative imaging and endoscopy are necessary to clarify the anatomical structure and guide surgical decision [6].

12.7 Follow-Up

Follow-up in gynecology is necessary during childbearing age, providing some help about childbearing guidance and vigilance against urinary system infection induced by sexual life. Pay attention to renal protection. Ultrasound examination of bladder and kidney is recommended during follow-up.

References

1. Peña A, Kessler O. Posterior cloaca: a unique defect. J Pediatr Surg. 1998;33(3):407–12.
2. Thomas D. The embryology of persistent cloaca and urogenital sinus malformations. Asian J Androl. 2020;22(2):124–8.
3. Wang Y, Hu S, Wang H. Multimodal ultrasound imaging of persistent urogenital sinus with uterus didelphys and double vagina malformation: a case report. Medicine (Baltimore). 2021;100(52):e28477.
4. Abouzeid AA, Mohammad SA, Shokry SS, et al. Posterior cloaca: a urogenital rather than anorectal anomaly. J Pediatr Urol. 2021;17(3):410.e1-.e7.
5. Ashour K, Shehata S, Osheba A. Cystourethroscopy versus contrast studies in urogenital sinus and cloacal anomalies in children. J Pediatr Surg. 2018;53(2):313–5.
6. Wood RJ, Reck-Burneo CA, Levitt MA. Cloacal malformations: technical aspects of the reconstruction and factors which predict surgical complexity. Front Pediatr. 2019;7:240.

GPSR Compliance

The European Union's (EU) General Product Safety Regulation (GPSR) is a set of rules that requires consumer products to be safe and our obligations to ensure this.

If you have any concerns about our products, you can contact us on ProductSafety@springernature.com

In case Publisher is established outside the EU, the EU authorized representative is:

Springer Nature Customer Service Center GmbH
Europaplatz 3
69115 Heidelberg, Germany

Batch number: 10732107

Printed by Printforce, the Netherlands